EVOLUTIONARY EATING™

How We Got Fat
and
7 Simple Fixes

Theresa Nesbitt, MD

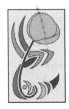

Praeclarus Press, LLC
www.PraeclarusPress.com

Praeclarus Press, LLC
2504 Sweetgum Lane
Amarillo, Texas 79124 USA
806-367-9950
www.PraeclarusPress.com

DISCLAIMER

The information contained in this publication is advisory only and is not
intended to replace sound clinical judgment or individualized patient care. The
author disclaims all warranties, whether expressed or implied, including any
warranty as the quality, accuracy, safety, or suitability of this information for any
particular purpose.

ISBN: 978-1-939807-052

Cover Design: Cornelia G. Murariu & Ken Tackett

Developmental Editing: Kathleen Kendall-Tackett

Copy Editing: Kathleen Kendall-Tackett & Amber Waller

Layout & Design: Cornelia G. Murariu

Logo design: Mohamad Sany Misnan

Illustrations: Roberto Osiris da Silva Filho

Operations: Scott Sherwood

ACKNOWLEDGEMENTS

I wish to express my sincere appreciation to all of my clients, friends and family for their extended long-term support. I owe particular thanks to my BrainChanging partner, Conor Hughes. Without his input and perspective, I would still be struggling to complete this book.

*"To my mother,
Agnes Heisley, who taught me
the value of the family meal."*

TABLE OF CONTENTS

CHAPTER 6

CHAPTER 7

CHAPTER 8

Evolutionary Eating

*"For most of human history, and
long before diets or gyms were invented,
women maintained a relatively slim
and shapely silhouette throughout their
adulthood. In the last 50 years, there has
been a dramatic change; not in our genes,
but in our environment.*

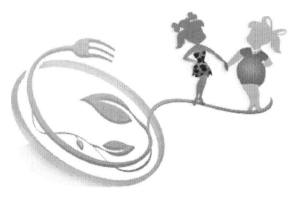

Evolutionary Eating *is your
quick and easy guide through the
fat traps of the modern world."*

Navigate This Book
Like a Buffet...Pace Yourself!

Unlike plants, which are able to make their own food, all animals must have an eating strategy. For most of the creatures on earth the eating strategy develops evolutionarily in concert with the local environment or habitat. Animals eat primarily by instinct.

Evolution endows individual species with characteristics that allow them to survive...anteaters have long tongues, hyenas have strong jaws to crack marrow bones left by lions, and gorillas have great big fermentation vats in their bellies to break down fibrous leaves, and free up nutrients.

Humans' evolutionary gift is a large brain. Brains are expensive, in evolutionary terms,.They require special nutrients, lots of calories, and they are very vulnerable to damage from lack of oxygen or glucose.

We humans are supposed to use our brains to learn how to choose and prepare foods so that they give us maximal nutritional benefit with minimal effort. For millions of years childhood represented the long period of time needed for individual humans to learn from their parents and community how to feed themselves and their families.

Now, food producers make enormous quantities of readily prepared, easily consumed, relatively inexpensive food that requires minimal effort.

Human beings evolved to adapt to almost any habitat, but never before on earth has food been so abundant. Generally it takes years to "learn how to eat," and this book attempts to cover a lot of useful strategies in a couple hundred pages.

I recommend you adopt the "buffet strategy"

Buffets are overwhelming for unskilled eaters. There are too many choices and everything looks good. Our brains start sending out messages like a roomful of unruly children to eat that, and that, and THAT!

You can't learn the skills of eating by gorging on information. You have to choose and digest strategies one at a time. Some strategies will be easy and appealing...so try them first. Some strategies you might never try, or perhaps you will give them a try and pass.

Approach the book as you would a buffet

Survey what is available. Read through the book to get an overall sense. Don't start trying out things as soon as you see them. Use a small plate. You can always go back for more. Focus on one concept at a time. Only put two items on your plate at one time. Learning a new skill requires more than knowledge...it requires practice or many repetitions before it becomes habit. Try and limit yourself to two new skills a week. Start by changing your environment. This is much easier and more effective than changing your behavior.

Habitats make habits. Rather than resist temptation, it's better to avoid it by making your personal space less tempting and stressful.

Avoid the buffet, or at least turn your back on it. Focus on making your personal space, a sanctuary, where you are not continuously bombarded with cues to eat.

Evolutionary Eating

PROLOGUE

*"Many unskilled eaters are
at the mercy of the hormonal horrors
that plague them with hunger pangs
around the clock. Here's a short
and humorous guide to conquering
all those demons once and for all!"*

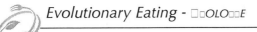

Haunted by Hunger?
How to Keep Your Demons at Bay!

Life can be a nightmare when you try to negotiate the modern food environment without the fundamental skills of eating. Millions of men and women spend hours each and every day tortured by "the food demons."

Food preoccupation, incessant cravings, and out-of-control binges don't come out of nowhere—they are the result of our confused brains signaling us to eat. Do the following scenarios sound familiar? Are you plagued by one or more of these demons?

The Zombie

A tendency to overeat in the evening usually indicates a problem with the fat-regulating hormone, leptin. When the sun begins to set, ravening, mindless hunger takes over. It can begin on the way home from work, or in the restless hours after dinner. Leptin 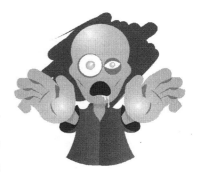 is what compels people to stare into the refrigerator, rifle through the cabinets, hit the streets for a fast food "fourth meal," or zone out in front of the television set with a bag of chips or bowls of ice cream. The following morning, you have a food hangover—filled with remorse and probably some undigested food. That evening demon is a Zombie—a creature of insatiable appetite with no frontal lobe function. It isn't a virus—this feeding frenzy is brought on by problems with the hormone leptin.

The Vampire

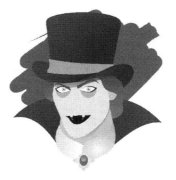

When the alarm clock starts buzzing, it's hard to drag yourself out of bed. Between guilt feelings about yesterday's indiscretions and general fatigue, skipping breakfast can seem like a good idea. It isn't!

One of the reasons people wake up without an appetite is because of problems with the hormone ghrelin. Ghrelin is produced by the stomach, and is associated with daily body rhythms, helping you to know that it is time to eat. If your stomach's growling, it's probably ghrelin.

People who don't get enough sleep, looking at bright light from their computer screens, or supersized television sets long into the evening hours, trick the body into thinking it's summertime—time to gorge and store fat in anticipation of winter. Eating regular meals—especially breakfast—helps regulate your hormones and get them working for you, rather than against you. You may say that you don't have time in the morning, but according to *Women's Health* magazine, the average American woman spends 54 minutes showering, dressing, doing her hair, and putting on her makeup each morning—and only five minutes on breakfast. When ghrelin is working well, you are hungry at mealtime, but not the rest of the time.

Appropriate ghrelin secretion depends on adequate nighttime sleep. When you snooze, you lose (weight). It also requires appropriate and consistent mealtime programming—and that means breakfast. Vampires don't function well in the daytime, and neither do many people struggling with their weight. If your appetite for breakfast is broken, the Vampire ghrelin is a likely culprit.

The Blob

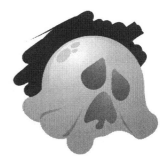

Unfortunately, there are worse things than skipping breakfast. Making the wrong food choices at breakfast time can awaken the Blob.

The Blob is an alien life form that consumes everything in sight. It made its movie debut in 1958, about the same time the processed-food industry took over the morning meal. The

Blob is the hormone insulin, and it needs a constant supply of food. While we are sleeping (and not eating), the Blob goes to sleep as well. But if you grab a quick breakfast that contains sugar or starch, the Blob will roar to life. Many unenlightened eaters have some of the Blob's favorite foods at breakfast— cereal, juice, muffins, pancakes, fat-free yogurt, toast, or bagels.

If you do, the Blob will be bossing you around for the rest of the day. That's because insulin is the hormone of fat storage. If too much insulin remains in your system, insulin resistance develops.

Under these circumstances, everything you eat is stuffed into your fat cells "for later," leaving you hungry even if you have just eaten.

The Blob will eat anything and everything. If you snack, or eat too many carbohydrates, you will have to battle it every day, and the Blob will always win.

The Banshee

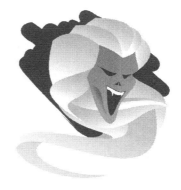

Once the day gets rolling, you may notice a persistent screaming in your ear. That's the Banshee. She's there to let you know that you are feeling a lot of stress.

Stress hormones, like cortisol and adrenaline, make you feel like you must do something immediately. Unskilled eaters usually shut the Banshee up by giving her something to eat—she can't scream with her mouth full.

Back in the olden days, when we felt stressed, we took a "coffee break." Then we decided coffee break meant coffee cake. The Banshee loves coffee cake (and vending machines).

When you handle stress with food, don't expect the Banshee to go away. As soon as she finishes eating, she'll be back—screaming just as loudly as ever.

The Ghost

Look at the time…it's 1:00 already… Did you eat lunch or did you just throw down some food to keep the demons at bay?

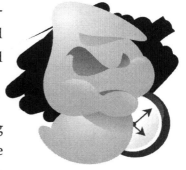

You haven't eaten a thing all day??? You probably have eaten—you just don't remember.

That's the Ghost, that invisible creature that wafts around, taking a bite here, and a nibble there. However, all those bites add up; if you eat like a Ghost, you will need a sheet to cover yourself up because your pants will (mysteriously) keep getting too tight.

The Pusher

Many unskilled eaters can make it through most of the day pretty well. They are often on a diet, so they eat a very carefully controlled breakfast, lunch, and snack.

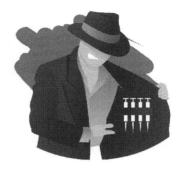

But when their energy begins to flag in the afternoon—that's when the Pusher pounces. This drug dealer doesn't dispense heroin and cocaine, but he does deal in two other white powders that hijack the exact same neurotransmitters.

Ordinary wheat contains exomorphins, or opiate-like substances. If you eat a lot of pasta, cereal, or bakery items, you are going to suffer from withdrawal just like other narcotic addicts. Yes, it's true—your bagel has an opiate effect on the brain. It starts off with a gnawing sensation that gets stronger until you eat something that contains wheat.

Now, sugar acts much like cocaine in the brain; studies show that lab rats (animals that are very fond of cocaine, like rhesus monkeys, will self-administer cocaine until they die) actually press a bar with greater enthusiasm and persistence for sugar than for cocaine. We can't ethically repeat this experiment on human beings, but watch people in front of the vending machine, pressing buttons for their Snickers bar… You get the idea. Unlike the withdrawal symptoms of wheat addiction, sugar is all about anticipation. It's distracting and causes a tremendous preoccupation with food. It becomes hard to think about anything else but your next fix. Drug dealer to the rescue! What's it going to be today?

Those low-fat packaged sweet treats work the same way. The Pusher, a.k.a., the food industry, knows the way to get a life-long customer is keep the cost low and the addictive quality high. That's what keeps their clients coming back for more.

The Witch

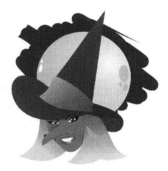

Women are especially suscep-tible to the Witch. At first, they think the Witch is their friend. She offers helpful constructive criticism that helps them stick to their diet.

She may say things like, "You really don't want to eat that—remember swimsuit season is just around the corner." But it doesn't take long for the Witch to turn into a real bitch. The messages become vicious and personal: "fat slob," "disgusting," "repulsive." A recent survey in *Glamour* magazine found that the average woman has 13 negative body thoughts a day, about one for every waking hour. Sadly, some women confess to having 50—or even 100—hateful thoughts about their body shape on a daily basis. That inner voice is the Witch, who is calculating and cruel. The Witch, being female, prefers to act indirectly. She gets you to overeat by stripping you of your defenses, so you are more susceptible to other forces of evil, like the Banshee, Blob, Zombie, and Werewolf.

The Werewolf

The Witch's favorite accomplice is her demon lover, the Werewolf.

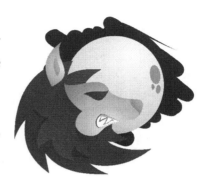

Werewolves in movies appear when the moon is full.

The Werewolf that sabotages your eating also comes out at a specific time—when you go on a restrictive diet.

Traditional diets are an attempt to keep the Werewolf under lock and key.

But diets are really flimsy things, and when the beast gets hungry enough, he will always break free. Once he gets loose, there is no stopping him until his enormous appetite is satisfied.

Unskilled eaters try to keep the beast at bay by counting calories and starving themselves. It doesn't work—when that Werewolf escapes, he is going on a huge binge.

The Barbarian

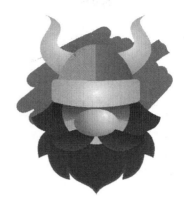

The boys tend to be less susceptible to the Witch than the girls. They think the Witch is a bitch, and they just ignore her. Males call their muffin tops "love handles." But the fellows aren't allowed to get off scot-free. Enter the testosterone-fueled Barbarian.

The Barbarian thinks it's manly to eat an entire bucket of fried chicken, or drink bucketloads of beer. Even worse, he is likely to poke fun at men who are struggling in the battle of the bulge. It's "girly" to be on a diet.

The Barbarian can be a real bully, and because he adores oversized, manly portions, he is a formidable foe. The Barbarian will tell you that you just need to exercise more.

Unfortunately, between the beer buzz, and the carbohydrate coma, you probably won't feel much like exercising… Maybe tomorrow.

The whole chamber of horrors

As night approaches, demons become more active and persistent:

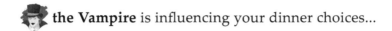 **the Vampire** is influencing your dinner choices...

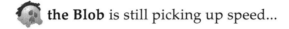 **the Blob** is still picking up speed...

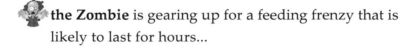 **the Zombie** is gearing up for a feeding frenzy that is likely to last for hours...

your afternoon sugar fix is wearing off...and your **Pusher** will deliver...

the **Banshee** isn't screaming, but she still won't shut up, a glass of wine—or three—will usually put her to bed for the night (She also likes that zoned-out feeling in front of the television.)

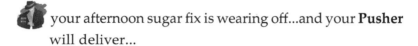 **the Ghost** will swear he hasn't eaten all day, you deserve a big dinner...

that bitch, **the Witch**, will fade into the shadows. She has already sown the seeds of havoc. But don't worry; she will be back tomorrow to remind you of all of your shortcomings...

Banish the demons instead of battling them!

That is what every day is like for unskilled eaters. Everyone has his or her own personal demons, but it isn't unusual for people struggling with their weight to be battling multiple demons every day. Here's the problem—very few of us are Vampire slayers or Blob blasters.

The solution isn't to battle the demons and win. The solution is to banish the demons and keep them at bay. The solution isn't to fight temptation; it's to avoid temptation. You don't need weapons like silver bullets, wooden stakes, or magical incantations. What you need is to become a competent eater…an eater who has mastered the basic skills of eating.

How do these skills help? They stop you from being such an easy target. Skill building takes time and practice, but it gives you solid and reliable protection against the forces of evil. You learn how to "keep out the demons."

Once they learn that you are no longer vulnerable, they will stop tormenting you. Not only will your weight normalize, but you will be able to eat until you are satisfied, and not think about food until it's time for your next meal.

You will be able to reclaim the evening, gradually unwinding until it is time to sleep, and awaken rested, refreshed, and ready for the day.

PREFACE

"Probably the most important skill every human must learn is the skill of eating."

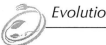

How Your Cinderella Story Can Have a Happily Ever After...

Everyone knows the tale of Cinderella, the beautiful princess trapped in a life of endless drudgery until she gets an unexpected visit from her fairy godmother.

Cinderella gets a makeover, complete with swank transportation, and is whisked off to the ball, where the handsome prince falls madly in love with her. Her glimpse of the happy life, though, is brief.

At the stroke of midnight, she finds herself back in her pile of cinders (in other words, hell). The prince looks everywhere for the gorgeous creature he fell in love with, but when he sees her covered in soot and sweat, he doesn't recognize her—his lovely was LOVELY. Eventually, though, he realizes she must be the one when she squeezes her foot into the unyielding, shows-every-flaw glass slipper.

Sounds like a parable for today's everyone's-desperate-to-lose-weight times, right? Well, yes—and no, too. Our stories aren't true Cinderella stories because we have the wrong goal. Cinderella's goal wasn't to fit into the glass slipper, and have the prince fall madly in love with her. Her goal was to live happily ever after.

We, however, live in a "once upon a time," in which we believe the answer to our problems is to squeeze into those new pants. We have figured out ways to transform our bodies temporarily—not with the help of a fairy godmother, but with the latest and greatest diet. Yet somehow, the midnight hour always catches up with us, and we find ourselves back in the same situation.

We don't live in fairyland; we live in FATland, surrounded by signals to eat, and an abundant supply of cheap, tasty food. The only thing that's "magic" is that food can be in your stomach literally seconds after you think about eating it.

We are only human—and humans are the naturally fattest species on Earth, fatter than hippos or polar bears. We have ten times the number of fat cells expected for mammals of our size. This distinctive feature evolved, along with our big human brains, to ensure that we had a constant supply of fuel, even when food became scarce.

Our brains need a continuous supply of oxygen; we breathe continuously because there is no air-storage tank. We eat intermittently because we do have a fat-storage tank—our adipose tissue.

The modern world is a very fat habitat. Humans haven't evolved into a new species in the last two million years; we have evolved into a highly adaptable one. We can live and thrive in a wide variety of environments, where we use our brains to develop the skills needed to nourish our bodies.

The modern world is triggering changes in our bodies that make us store and hoard fat. It is very difficult to "lose weight" in fat-storage mode, and even harder to keep it off. We aren't designed to lose weight, but rather to USE weight. So that's the real world. Those are the facts. But don't despair—not living in fairyland doesn't mean you can't make your dreams come true.

You don't need to be Cinderella to have a happily ever after, and you certainly don't need a prince to rescue you. Princes (doctors, fitness gurus, and diet experts) offer instant solutions, but these promises are illusory and empty. We all have an inborn weight-regulating mechanism, but we still must learn and use skills to master our current environment.

That might sound challenging, scary, or confusing, but don't worry, you will have help. Just think of me as your personal fairy godmother, and let's get working on that personal happily ever after—an attractive, healthy body that will last a lifetime.

INTRODUCTION

"In the modern world, where food is available anytime and anywhere, many adults have mastered the skills of dieting, but have yet to learn how to eat."

Why Skill Power Beats Willpower

"Have you heard about the diet that
makes you burn fat while you sleep?"

"I just got my hands on the newest fat-burning program.
It promises to shed the fat in just three minutes
and 46 seconds a day!"

"Well, I just got this new scientifically approved
weight-loss pill. It's guaranteed to take off
35 pounds in 30 days!"

Weight Loss. We all want it, and we all think we know how to get it. Diets, Pills, Exercise, Surgery...they all work...right? I thought they did too, but that was before I heard all of the above comments from the same client.

Sarah was always on the latest and greatest fat-burning, fat-shedding, weight-loss program. The problem for her, and everybody else, was that it was just impossible to stick to any of those "fat-burning miracles" forever.

Although various weight-loss programs differ, most of them place an emphasis on the same underlying factor: CALORIES. How to regulate them. How to balance them. How to burn them off.

Wanna lose weight? It's easy, you just:

Eat less.

Move more.

Take this pill.

Have it surgically removed.

OR

Wish for a fairy godmother who can instantly transform
your shape from round pumpkin to sleek hourglass.

These concepts have been around for some time now, and are still the most commonly used methods for weight loss. But do they actually work? Let's take a look...

Why not diet...more, harder, better?

Dieting is the most common of the weight-loss strategies. Many of us have had the giddy experience of watching the numbers go down on the scale, buying new clothes in a smaller size, and getting lots of compliments on our successful weight loss.

If you are like 98% of the population, the results don't last longer than a year or two. Even for those who continue to diet and exercise, the weight usually comes back, often much more quickly than it was lost.

Over time, each diet becomes more and more difficult. The weight refuses to budge despite more desperate calorie restriction. Any loss of control leads to further weight gain, along with feelings of shame, depression, and hopelessness.

This lasts until the next new diet, the one that will finally work. The reality is that if these diets did work there would not be thousands of diet and weight-loss programs; there would be one. So if diets don't work…

Why not exercise more, harder, better?

Ah-ha! Exercise makes sense. You know, the whole calories-in, calories-out thing.

Well, before you sign up for yet another gym membership, let's take a quick look at the stats. The National Weight Control Registry is an American membership platform that was developed to identify the characteristics of individuals who have succeeded at long-term weight loss.

To be eligible to join the registry, you must have lost at least 30 pounds, and maintained that weight loss for at least one year. In studies done on these successful dieters, one particular finding stands out. Out of all the successful registrants, only 1% relied on exercise alone to maintain their weight.

This may seem like a better percentage than the diet method; however, this is a percentage of successful weight-loss campaigns, and doesn't account for the hundreds of thousands of people who try exercise and fail. An active lifestyle is associated with long-term weight maintenance, but it's hard to know which comes first. It's a lot more fun to move around when you are 100 pounds lighter.

41

Exercise alone, even running marathons, isn't likely to help you get where you want to go. In 1989, Danish researchers had obese men and women spend 18 months training for a marathon. After a year and a half, the men had shed just five pounds, and the women had lost no weight whatsoever. So if you thought dieting was ineffective, exercise, especially for women, has even poorer results. That burn you're feeling isn't fat–it's the dollars in your wallet and the hours in your day. Not to worry. Instead...

Why not take weight-loss pills?

"Take this pill and your troubles will be gone forever!" We all wish that there was a pill for everything.

A pill that puts a million dollars in your bank account? I'd buy that. A pill that could make you fly? I'd buy that too! Pills that can make you lose weight and keep it off forever? Sign me up! It is this illusion of the magic diet pill that has caused an explosion in the pharmacological industry, and although pills don't work (or at least safe ones don't), people keep buying them. Let's take a brief look at the history of diet pills.

The most "successful" weight-loss pill in history was actually a combination of two drugs—phentermine and fenfluramine, more commonly known as phen-fen. Phen-fen acted in a complex way on two brain chemicals, serotonin and dopamine, and reduced the reward that people would seek from food. So why is phen-fen not available today? It was pulled off the market in 1997 because it produced serious, and sometimes life-threatening, cardiac side effects. Not to worry, though, when all else fails…

Why not remove it?

Ah, surgery. It's a drastic measure, but one with potentially dramatic results. Whether it's liposuction, tummy-tucks, or Brazilian butt lifts, the allure of instant results with no effort has resulted in our spending well over a billion dollars a year on surgical body sculpting. None of these surgeries are cheap, and few are covered by insurance. They would probably be even more popular if they were.

But here's biggest the problem with them: even when you suck the extra fat out and throw it away, you haven't changed the fact that many of the overweight patients are hormonally in fat-storage mode. They are gaining weight, and just trying to keep pace. It's like bailing water out of a leaky boat, and going nowhere—you are stuck bailing and bailing until someone comes along to rescue you.

Because liposuction doesn't change behavior, we find ourselves "still in the same boat." After the surgery, most people will continue the same behaviors that made them fat in the first place, so it always comes back. For those who are morbidly obese and metabolically broken, there is gastric bypass or lap-band surgery, very invasive last-ditch efforts for those who feel they have no other option.

Even if the surgery is "successful," there are severe side effects that last a lifetime. Even more troubling is the risk of death, either during the surgery or later in life. It's not a happy ending at all.

I'm pretty sure I know what you're thinking right about now: *"Thanks for ruining my day, Doc! If these methods don't work, then what does?" What Else is There!?"*

Well, first of all, there is relief. And happiness. You should be happy in the knowledge that the reason you can't get to and remain at the weight you want is not because you are inadequate, or that you don't have "sufficient willpower."

The methods you have been using are the real failures— they just don't work. So when you try dieting, or weight loss, or pills, or surgery, you are not addressing the underlying reason that you have excess fat. You are treating the symptoms, not the system, so you've lost the game before you've even begun.

What I am about to tell you is probably something that you have never heard before, and it is the same thing I told Sarah when she came to see me.

Forget about these methods. They all address the symptom—excess fat—but none of them address the SYSTEM, which is the reason why you are fat in the first place. The real reason you are fat is that...

You don't know how to eat!

Yes, that's right. You don't know how to eat. Most people don't realize that eating is an acquired skill, not one we are born with.

When we come into the world, we have legs, but can't walk; we have hands, but we can't write; and we have mouths, but can't talk. In the same way, we need food, but we don't know how to eat. Just as we learn to walk, talk, and write, we must also learn to eat.

If you are overweight, you have a food preoccupation. If you are a yo-yo dieter, you are constantly on weight-loss programs. If you are always monitoring what you put in your mouth…it's not because there is something wrong with you. It's because you haven't learned the skills of eating. You aren't "broken," and you don't need "fixing." All you need is skill. You aren't born with skills; you must learn them.

When asked to name a genius, the most common answer is Albert Einstein. Einstein was asked how he would save the world if he only had 60 minutes to do it. He answered: *"If I had an hour to save the world, I would spend 59 minutes defining the problem and one minute finding solutions."* I think this can be rewritten to address our current situation. I'd like to call it the problem with the problem. And let's call this the solution book.

We are all looking for the solution to keeping off weight, but what good is a solution if it's addressing the wrong problem? That's what the current weight-loss strategies all do.

Obesity isn't the actual problem. Obesity is, in fact, a predictable result of ignorant humans living in an obesogenic environment—that is to say, "the modern world."

The reason that every single weight-loss strategy is bound to fail is that they are all based on the skills of weight loss, but none of them teach the skills of eating. Weight-loss skills help you with weight loss, but there is only so much weight that you can lose. Eating disorders are not a "successful outcome."

So if you are fortunate and your short-term weight-loss strategy gets you to your desired weight, then what? When we loosen up on the restrictive diet, most of us slide back to our old eating habits, either slowly or quickly.

For most people, the problem is compounded because while they were on their restrictive-reducing program, they remained hormonally in fat-storage mode.

When your body is in fat-storage mode, the default is slow, but steady weight gain. This goes on for a while until something jars you into action—an unkind remark, a special occasion, or a closet full of clothes that don't fit. When you restrict your food intake you can "lose weight," but your hormonal status doesn't change... you are still in fat-storage mode. As soon as they give up struggling to "lose weight," the pounds will come back.

And statistics show that you usually end up heavier than before. The real problem isn't that you don't know how to diet. The problem is that you haven't learned the skills of eating. Until you learn those skills, you will always be struggling.

This book—*Evolutionary Eating: How We Got Fat & 7 Simple Fixes*—will introduce you to each of the skills that you need to become a competent eater. Every chapter will outline a problem, and then address it with one of the skills of eating. There are also 10 to 15 quick-start strategies at the end of each chapter to really get you going.

Evolutionary Eating: How We Got Fat & 7 Simple Fixes is a little like boot camp, or perhaps more accurately, "booty" camp. Boot camp takes a bunch of kids and gives them enough skill to enter enemy territory, and hopefully avoid the worst of the danger. But a graduate of boot camp is still a raw recruit, not a seasoned soldier.

This book is designed to introduce you to the fundamental skills of eating. Though it will take many months to develop expertise, if you practice the suggested behaviors, you will develop eating competence.

The modern world is a dangerous place for unskilled eaters interested in staying thin and healthy. It is full of temptations and has no boundaries—it's like Pleasure Island from *Pinocchio*.

Everywhere we look, we are offered food forgeries—synthetic foods—that are very confusing to our natural weight-regulating mechanism. The media sends us hundreds of irresistible marketing messages each day promising that these "foods" are quick, economical, delicious, and even healthy.

They're not healthy. They are saboteurs. And it's our job to learn to avoid them.

Willpower has its limitations. Skill power is what is required to navigate the modern food environment. That is what this book—and I—want to teach you.

Let's get going!

CHAPTER 1

"The modern world is fat-provoking;
without skills and strategies,
you are always going to be gaining,
rather than maintaining."

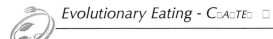

Why We Got Fat and How to Fix It

All humans learn how to eat. We don't think about it—it happens automatically when we observe and adopt the eating habits of the people around us—family, friends, and even the people we see on television.

Our brains are also designed to respond to cues from the world around us. The sights and smells of food are likely to trigger signals to eat, signals that are reinforced when we respond to the impulses, just like your puppy is more likely to keep begging if you always give him treats.

The world is full of treats, but woefully lacking in either training or restraining (which, by the way, is not the same as restricting). As a result, we are always gaining. What you gain, you have to lose. All of which has gotten us to where we are now—to becoming a society that believes winning the title of "biggest loser" is an appropriate goal.

All diet and weight-loss programs do exactly what they say they do...make you lose weight. For most people, that is ample confirmation that these programs are the solution to any weight and excess-fat problems. That's the trap. Diet and weight-loss programs are designed to help you lose weight, but fail to address the real problem, which is that we don't have a clue about how to stop over-accumulating.

A woman who experiences pain whenever she puts weight on her foot might decide to use crutches. This will be a good temporary strategy if she has a sprained ankle. But what if the reason for the pain is a sharp pebble in her shoe? If she uses the crutches, the pain will go away, but as soon as she begins walking normally, it will return.

This is what happens when we go on calorie-restricting diets. We use a weight-loss strategy of "losing weight" instead of repairing our eating habits. We are leaving our eating habits to chance, like someone who is running blind over rough and unfamiliar terrain—someone who will keep spraining her ankle.

Why do we keep repeating such behavior when it's not getting us where we want to go?

The unfortunate reality is that we are all human, and our default strategy is to do what everyone around us is doing. The modern world is fat-provoking; without skills and strategies, you are always going to be gaining rather than maintaining. If your diet is successful, you might lose all the weight—maybe you can drop a few sizes, or go from 180 pounds to your target weight of 130. But now what?

In order to "lose weight," you most likely restricted your calories, eliminated a lot of "bad foods," and engaged in some type of fat-burning exercise. When you attained your desired weight, you probably got a lot of compliments, encouragement, and maybe even a new wardrobe. Now, you have to switch your goal to maintaining. But what does that mean?

In theory, post "diet" weight maintenance means that if you ease up on your dietary restrictions, your weight loss will level off, and you will remain at your target weight.

In reality, however, this feat is quite difficult to accomplish—it's probably easier to balance on the head of a pin than to hold the needle of the scale steady by using the "diet lite" approach. The reality is that if you really knew how to avoid "regaining the weight," you would have never needed to diet in the first place.

The diet-and-weight-loss industry provides products and services. These companies aren't interested in becoming obsolete, which means we have placed all of our trust in people who have a vested interest.

When—and if—you reach your target weight, you must consider two things. The first is that you can't really lose much more weight. If you are at 130 pounds, then losing another 50 is either ludicrous or dangerous. The second is that even if you developed some "weight loss" skills, you still don't have "stop gaining skills," which is the underlying problem. When you are always gaining you have no choice but to keep trying to lose.

This, unfortunately, is where 99% of dieters find themselves. The behaviors needed to lose 50 pounds are not the same behaviors that will maintain your target weight.

But when you "stop dieting," you revert to a default position—and that default position is going to be fat-storage mode. Why? Because although you might be a very knowledgeable dieter; you haven't learned and practiced the fundamental skills of eating. The weight gain/weight loss cycle will continue because you haven't figured out that you need to get the pebble out of your shoe. Ask yourself what you are trying to achieve.

The average American lives to be almost 70. That's a lot of years, and a lot of cycles of weight gain and weight loss if you have the wrong goals—especially if you have the wrong TYPE of goals.

The way of life vs. the weigh of life

When you go on a diet, join a gym, or pay a personal trainer, you probably have result-based goals, which are measurable and describe exactly what you want to accomplish. An example of a results-based goal would be: "I want to lose 30 pounds in 30 days."

The big problem with results-based goals is that once you've reached your goal, you have nowhere to go but backwards. It's especially frustrating when you realize a single episode of "successful" weight loss can wreak long-term havoc on your weight management. How often do we say, "I can start my diet tomorrow"? The temptation to do this is multiplied when we tell ourselves "I've done it before—I can do it again."

If you have a goal like "lose 30 pounds in 30 days," you may very well accomplish it, but you will have learned nothing about the lifelong behaviors you need to maintain your "new" body. Once you lose the weight, you'll still be working off the faulty model of "lose 30 pounds in 30 days."

The only way you can continue to achieve that goal is to regain the 30 pounds so that you can lose it again. Soon you are engaging in a constant battle of losing, gaining, losing, gaining, simply because you have a goal dictating that you do so.

In contrast, long-term change, which is really the only valuable kind, lends itself much better to behavioral goals than to results-based goals. It makes perfect sense…if you want to make a behavioral change, focus on behavioral goals. But it's the glistening shine of the instant gratification, results-based goal that often gets in our way of making such distinctions. One of my favorite ways to describe this to people is by explaining the true meaning of the word diet.

Diet stems from the Latin word *diaeta*, which means "prescribed way of life." If you wish to achieve a healthy weight and maintain that weight loss, this is the most important point of this entire book. *Changing your diet is not about calorie restriction, exercising more, or depriving yourself. Instead, changing your diet is about changing your "way of life."* And how do you change your life? You focus on the WAY, not on the WEIGH.

You must learn and practice behaviors that become lifetime habits. A habit, by definition, is a behavior that occurs without conscious thought, or effort. Until you understand this point, you will continue to search for that "secret diet plan," or the "supercharged exercise program" or the "new fat-loss pill."

But despite what people try to sell us, none of these work. A diet is not something that you are "on," it is something that you do. And the thing that we are supposed to do is to eat, not diet. Instead of becoming skillful dieters, we need to become skillful eaters.

If you are having trouble with your weight, it's not because there is something wrong with you, or that you lack willpower. In fact, you probably have immense willpower because dieting requires it.

Instead, the problem is simply that you don't know how to eat. When you go from 200 pounds to, say, 130 pounds, you have been successful in your goal of weight loss. But now how do you shift into weight maintenance? No weight-loss strategy can help you with this because every one of them focuses you on the wrong goals.

How can you expect a happily ever after when your goal is to fit into the glass slipper? Substitute the WAY of life diet for the WEIGH of life diet. In reality, you can't "lose" weight anyway. "Lose weight" is just a phrase we use because lose is the opposite of gain.

You certainly can gain weight, but our bodies are designed to balance out gaining and using weight (resulting in a stable weight over a lifetime). They are not designed to gain and lose weight in the yo-yo, fatty-skinny cycle, in which you will slowly and surely get a progressively fatter body while giving the fitness industry a fatter wallet.

Substitute the WAY OF LIFE diet for the WEIGH of life diet

When you go on a calorie-restricting or exercise program, and you monitor your progress by inches or pounds, you're going to see results, especially if you stick with it.

But inside of every person, there is a natural weight-regulating mechanism, and it's keeping track of everything. Every important function in your body is regulated to stay within a healthful range—your blood pressure, body temperature, and blood sugar are just a few examples.

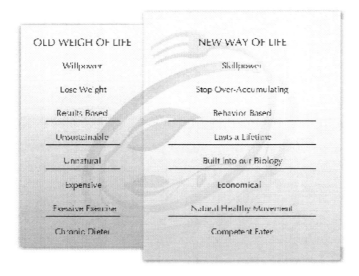

OLD WEIGH OF LIFE	NEW WAY OF LIFE
Willpower	Skillpower
Lose Weight	Stop Over-Accumulating
Results Based	Behavior Based
Unsustainable	Lasts a Lifetime
Unnatural	Built into our Biology
Expensive	Economical
Excessive Exercise	Natural Healthy Movement
Chronic Dieter	Competent Eater

Gary Taubes, the bestselling author of *Good Calories, Bad Calories* and *Why We Get Fat,* points out that our bodies are so exquisitely calibrated to regulate hunger—satiety—and fat storage that as little as a daily 20 calorie excess or deficit (just a single extra or absent bite of food) over time would push us into morbid obesity or starvation.

Survival functions are not left to chance, but it makes sense that if we "err," it will be on the side of a little extra body fat rather than too little. In fact, for females, too little body fat is the original birth control—your brain doesn't care how you look like naked, but it is definitely interested in whether you have enough body fat to grow a baby over a long winter when food is scarce.

Humans evolved along with cyclical seasons. For the millions of years humans existed on Earth, it was nature that dictated when there was feast and when there was famine. Our bodies are designed to adjust when nature makes food scarce or abundant.

About 10,000 years ago, humans, with their big brains, invented agriculture, which effectively reduced periods of famine by extending the growing season. But it's only been in about the past 100 years that we've learned how to prolong the feast with tasty prepared foods available to us at all times of the day (and night). One just needs to take a look at our rapidly expanding bodies, and the escalating problem of obesity in the next generation, to get the message...

It's not nice to fool mother nature!

When you decide to voluntarily feast and starve (indulge and diet), you activate sensitive monitors within your body designed to keep you alive. When you go on "a diet," particularly a more restrictive one, you reset your hormonal balance so that it becomes very vigilant in the future when it detects fewer calories in the environment.

When you initiate a new weight-loss regimen, your mind and your body are in general agreement—body fat can be used as fuel—you "use weight" and, according to the scale, you "lose weight."

But your body isn't just thinking about the size 8 dress you want to wear to your high school reunion. It is designed for survival first, and fertility second, which means hormonally you are going to trigger a number of fat-protecting mechanisms.

Your body is going to make it difficult for fat cells to release fat for fuel, your metabolism is going to downregulate, your baseline energy is going to drop, and your hunger and interest in food is going to increase. What that means is that instead of forming a healthy habit, you will have set yourself up to work—diligently and painfully—on weight loss every single day.

That is why this is such a poor long-term strategy. If you look at the one-year follow-ups of anyone who tries these weight-loss programs, most have gained the weight right back. If you look at three-year and five-year follow-ups, almost everybody has gained the weight back.

Now, contrast that with those who have been able to reach their desired figure and maintain that figure for a period of greater than five years. Not only have those people accomplished that, but they are also not obsessed with food.

The reason they have been able to change is not because of this or that diet, or this or that weight-loss method. They have been successful because they've undergone a complete lifestyle transformation.

These people were able to reset their weight-regulating mechanism so the weight they are now is the natural weight for their body. Dieting does the opposite; it disrupts your weight-regulating mechanism, so you are stuck with a fluctuating weight. To keep the weight off for good, you need to reset your weight-regulating mechanism to the weight that you want. The only way you can do that is by learning the fundamental skills of eating.

Socrates said the beginning of wisdom is the definition of terms. So, what is a skill?

A skill is something:
- You are not born knowing,
- You have to learn,
- You can always refine and improve,
- You must practice in order to become proficient, and
- That deteriorates if you neglect it or reject it.

And eating is a skill because:
- We aren't born with a great deal of eating knowledge; we only know that sweet tastes good, and that when food is available, you should eat until you can't eat anymore.

- Traditionally, human children have learned over a period of years what, when, where, and how to eat. We unconsciously adopt the eating habits of the people with whom we eat. These are the when, what, where, who, how, and why skills—the fundamental skills of eating that must be learned.

Because the environment is always changing, often becoming more challenging, we need our skills to keep up. Habitats make habits, to successfully navigate the "old country buffet," or to bypass the muffins in the break room, you need skill power, not willpower.

Evolutionary Eating is a set of skills; skills that can be learned

There is a reason why, despite the over 20,000 "weight loss" books on Amazon, we are getting fatter every year. Weight-loss books may make you more aware of your eating habits, and that's a start.

But permanently changing the way you think about food—and the way you consume it—requires action and practice. It requires a change in behavior. It's the difference between New Year's Resolutions and New Year's results. Resolutions are just words. New thinking, combined with action and practice (behavior), produces lasting results—not just for a year, but for a lifetime.

I don't think of *Evolutionary Eating: How We Got Fat & 7 Simple Fixes* as a weight-loss book. I think of it as a weight-management manual. Its goal—and mine—is to help you develop the skills necessary to become a competent eater. Over time, if you choose to enhance your skills, you can become an "elite" eater. That means that you can calmly and safely roam the hazardous terrain of donuts, drive-thrus, and "dinner is served," whenever and wherever. You will no longer act like a "kid in a candy shop" because you will have mastered the mature-adult skills.

When you practice the skills of eating until they become habit, your body will hormonally adjust, and you will no longer be locked in fat-storage mode. With a new goal of using weight (behavior-based), rather than losing weight (results-based), your normal physiologic weight-regulating mechanisms will keep your hunger and energy in a happy, healthy equilibrium. The biologic name for this condition is homeostasis.

When you achieve "homeostatic hum," you reap the rewards of a healthy, fit body. You get to say goodbye to clothing that grows progressively tighter, self-loathing for your "lack of self-discipline," and successive rounds of painful deprivation. Doesn't it make you want to scream "Freedom!?" Like Mel Gibson in *Braveheart?* Well, go ahead and scream: *Freedom!* That's a start. We've done the thinking—but now we have to do the real work: the doing. It is time to begin changing our behavior by practicing the fundamental skills of eating.

Let's go!

Change From Results-Based Goals to Behavior-Based Goals

It's not enough to change your mind, but doing so is the first step in the right direction. When you change your mindset, you start on the path that takes you where you want to go.

Practice, practice, practice

Habit isn't just a word; we have to practice a new behavior over and over for it to become a habit. As you do so, you strengthen connections in your brain, which makes them start to operate faster and more efficiently. The brain and the nervous system are composed of wired and wireless connections, just like your home environment.

Developing a habit is like insulating the wires, or increasing the bandwidth. We used to think the adult brain wasn't capable of changing, but the new research on neuroplasticity has demonstrated that although brain cells don't change much, brain connections can change a lot.

Train smarter, not harder

You probably don't think of it this way, but when you practice a new behavior in order to increase your skill, you are training yourself. That's why I think of *Evolutionary Eating* as a training manual. You could train hard and get results but, over time, most people who do so tend to get exhausted or bored. That's what happens when people willpower instead of skill power. Willpower is very effective, but it doesn't last long. Training smart means you are using willpower wisely.

Using your willpower to change your habitat, not your habits, is an example of using willpower wisely. When you put effort into structuring your environment, changes in behavior are unconscious, and therefore effortless and painless.

No pain, no gain

When you train smart, with behavioral-based goals, you avoid the pain of an unattractive, unhealthy body, and the torture of traditional weight-loss regimens. Because when there is "no gain," there is no need to lose!

Most people have results-based weight goals. For instance, Jane might think, "I want to go from weighing 150 pounds to 120, and I want to maintain this weight for the rest of my life." One problem with this mindset is that pounds are just numbers on a scale. Really, what Jane wants is to look a certain way, so she (and you) should be thinking hourglass, not scale. But that isn't the biggest problem. The real flaw with Jane's thinking is that her goal isn't focused on behavior.

So what are behavioral-based goals? Basically, behavioral-based goals are the things we need to change in order to achieve the lifelong results we want. When we have behavioral goals, we are working on our habits. We need to target the behaviors that have a significant impact on our long-term weight management.

In this book, I categorize the behaviors into the fundamental skills of eating—the when, what, where, who, how, and why skills. Note that the skills of eating are based upon behaviors, not results.

A behavior is something that you can do which, if you practice it often, becomes an automatic stress-free habit that lasts a lifetime. Results are never life-long; you can't continue to lose 30 pounds for the rest of your life! This means that the behaviors you might have been implementing in the past to lose those 30 pounds are actually useless in the long term because you simply can't sustain them!

Restricting your eating is painful. Restraining your eating, on the other hand, is at first mildly uncomfortable, and then mindlessly familiar and comfortable. For comparison, let's consider something else we train by restraining: potty habits.

Human beings aren't born potty-trained. For the first few years of life, we go whenever, and wherever we feel like it. Somewhere in toddlerhood, our parents and guardians train us to restrain from going potty in places other than the toilet. It's uncomfortable at first for the child, yet most adults don't really feel restricted by having to get up from the sofa during a television commercial to go to the bathroom. That is restraint.

Restriction, on the other hand, means denying really physiological urges. If you drink a gallon of iced tea, and then can't find a restroom, you are going to be more than a little uncomfortable. The mind can amplify this signal, just like it does for eating.

As soon as you realize that you "can't go," especially if you don't know when you will be able to relieve yourself, it's impossible to think of anything else. In the same way, when you restrict food and tell yourself you "can't eat," you can't think about anything else but food.

It's a much better strategy to decide when and where you are going to eat, and make sure doing so is possible. That way you never have to tell yourself you are "not eating"; instead, you are always saying, "I can eat at that time or that place. For now, I can wait."

What's my—and your—strategy?

According to *Webster's*, a strategy is a plan or method for achieving a particular goal, usually over a long period of time. A tactic is an action or strategy designed to achieve a certain end. In this book, I focus on strategies because they are long-term, behavioral-based plans for achieving a stable weight that lasts a lifetime (the Peace Plan), as opposed to short-term, result-based tactics to achieve a certain specific outcome— lose 30 pounds in 30 days (the Battle Plan).

By focusing on strategies, we develop foundational skills for ourselves that can be built on and refined for life. The more you practice a skill, the easier and more automatic it becomes; as many people like to say, "Practice makes perfect." I prefer to say "Practice makes permanent"—because only perfect practice makes perfect. Pursuit of perfection is stressful and overrated.

If you are skill building from the ground up, you might as well adopt the point of view that "good enough" will serve as today's "perfect." Really, you have the rest of your life to keep improving. Through research in skill building, I have learned that it is crucial to have a framework—an intentional reason for practice.

Daniel Coyle investigated skill building extensively in his groundbreaking book, *The Talent Code: Greatness Isn't Born, It's Grown, Here's How*. Coyle found that there is a similar formula for greatness in many aspects of life. Academics, music, and sports are just a few examples.

He calls the formula a Deep Practice Model, and identifies these important characteristics of successful skill building.

1. Create a vision for what you are trying to achieve

This vision is the framework for the skill.

The *Evolutionary Eating* framework is to achieve and maintain a stable healthy weight for life.

2. Big skills are combinations of little skills

Quick-start strategies are loads of little skills that, over time, produce skillful and competent eating.

It's important to take action—use drills to build skills. Writing is a particularly effective action.

3. Practice, practice, and practice some more

This is the best way to let your brain prioritize. Rewiring brains requires significant effort. Practice makes it happen.

Every time you get a chance to practice a new behavior, you strengthen it.

Every time you practice an old undesirable behavior, you strengthen that too!

That's why it's important to devise drills that are a little challenging, but not too difficult or unpleasant.

Evolutionary Eating quick-start strategies, which appear at the end of every chapter, take a multifaceted approach and usually fall into one of the following categories:

Change your thoughts.

Change your actions.

Change your direction based upon new information, knowledge, and skills (assess and refine).

Before we move on to the next chapter, here are some Quick-Start Strategies to help you review and put into action what I've shared with you so far.

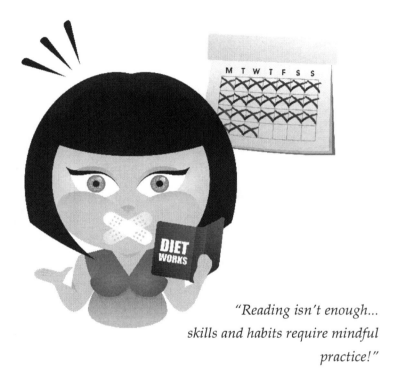

"Reading isn't enough...
skills and habits require mindful
practice!"

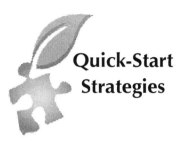

Quick-Start Strategies

1) Use skill power, NOT willpower

If you are using willpower to lose and maintain weight, it is only a matter of time before you relapse. Success at weight control is not about willpower. The definition of willpower is work, and continuing to rely on it is a heavy burden. Those who succeed at weight control do not have more willpower; they simply have better strategies.

There are so many factors that influence what you eat—your neurological hardwiring, your value system, your biology, advertising and marketing—that relying on willpower alone is disastrous. The most important factor for success is having strategies that work for you.

2) Make change your #1 priority

In reality, most people who try to lose weight don't really want to change. They think that losing weight is a good idea, and they think that being thinner is what they want but, sadly, these are only thoughts.

If you want to lose weight and maintain your weight loss, you must make it the number-one priority in your life.

All of life requires adjustments and tradeoffs. If you want to lose weight, there are things you will have to do that you probably won't want to.

Now is the time to stop resenting what you need to do to keep your body healthy. Everything else you value in your life—your career, your relationships, your children—has taken work, focus, and endurance. Weight loss is no different.

Succeeding in accomplishing your goal will require making this your number-one priority. Unless you do that, you will be dieting for the rest of your life. The good news is that once you make your diet a "way of life," maintaining a healthy weight will take much less effort. Remember, willpower won't work.

3) Don't get complacent

Possibly one of the biggest mistakes that a dieter can make is becoming complacent. You lose weight, you feel great, your clothes fit you better, and everybody is commenting on how good you look. As a reward, you decide to indulge in your favorite treat. No big deal, you've been so good up to now. Right?

Unfortunately, an indulgence like this leads to a second indulgence, and then to a third, until finally, in a few days, you will have undone all of your hard work. Remember, being thin is a lifestyle, and it is difficult to change your whole life in a few weeks. Change takes time, and just because you've lost weight doesn't mean you've lost vulnerability. It takes a long time to rewire the brain, and it is easy to slip back into old habits.

4) Stumbles are just setbacks, not strikeouts

Life is hard; food is easy. You are going to stumble and you might even fall. It isn't fatal. Get up and keep going. Realize that when the going gets rough, progress may be slow. There is no shame in plodding.

According to James O. Prochaska, John Norcross, and Carlo DiClemente, authors of the fantastic book, *Changing for Good,* the number-one indicator of successful change is never giving up on yourself.

Change takes massive effort and time, and it is highly unlikely that you will succeed at your first attempt. This does not mean that you should do the same thing over and over again. (That's the definition of insanity.) Instead, look for what works for you. Use the strategies in this book and figure out what suits your needs. What works for me or somebody else will not necessarily work for you. Continue to refine and improve, and most importantly, never give up.

5) Establish a routine

Your brain loves habits and routines, especially when it comes to food. Because food holds such high survival value, your brain is constantly evaluating where your next meal is coming from.

This is one of the main reasons why you may instantly feel hungry as soon as you see ice cream. Your brain knows that ice cream is high in fat and sugar—a great energy source—so it will tell you that you are hungry just because it is not sure that ice cream will be available in the near future. (Weird, I know!)

What is wonderful about this, however, is that if you can establish a consistent routine, your brain will restructure when it releases certain hunger hormones so you will only get hungry when it is time to eat. Reassure your brain that food is available by always eating at the same times, and your cravings will greatly decrease. One topic to which I'll return over and over is the importance of regularly scheduled meals in skill-building eating competence.

6) Eat breakfast

Study after study has shown that eating breakfast is associated with achieving and maintaining your ideal body weight, yet what is the most common meal skipped in the day? You guessed it. Breakfast!

Eating breakfast does a number of positive things, it raises your metabolism, provides you with energy so you are more likely to move during the day, prevents a blood sugar drop that would normally result in sugar cravings, and gives you a positive start to the day which, mentally, you will want to continue with your other meals.

Finally, people who skip breakfast are much more likely to overeat at dinner. So, the message is clear. Eat a good, healthy breakfast, and you will be more likely to maintain a healthy weight!

7) Restrain, don't restrict

Traditional diets are usually restrictive; you consume fewer calories by consciously eating smaller amounts, and prohibiting "fattening" foods.

Expert dieters often know the exact calorie count of thousands of food items; they may even know the magical formulas for glycemic index, carbohydrate chemistry, and food combining.

Expert eaters practice restraint, not restriction. They don't skip meals; they learn to eat enough at one meal to last until the next. They don't resist temptation, but sometimes they test it. Setting appropriate and bearable boundaries helps you fence out an overabundance of temptations.

8) Frame in

Are you more of a carrot or stick person? If you are motivated by positive experiences, perhaps you need to ramp up the frame. A frame is something that surrounds a beautiful and valued piece of art. An *Evolutionary-Eating* frame symbolically surrounds a valuable experience or behavior.

Frame in your meals—take time to sit and savor. Learn to look forward to eating opportunities. You don't need to eat on demand like an infant. When you restrain from eating between meals, you allow your body to develop knowledge and maturity.

Grandmas knew the old-time wisdom that snacks spoil your supper. Don't treat your eating experiences like bad graffiti or thoughtless doodles; frame in your meals or treats. If you want a sweet, then make it special.

9) Fence out

Many of us are more motivated by the stick, a well-known aspect of human psychology called negativity bias. We will often go to great lengths to avoid pain or even discomfort.

A useful "stick" strategy is to fence out. It's very painful and exhausting to constantly resist temptation. (In fact, there is an ancient Greek myth about the origin of the word "tantalize.") In order to avoid the pain of temptation, it's best to remove the object of temptation from your immediate surroundings. Out of site (and sight) may be out of might. Within reach and within sight is…torture. Build a tall, sturdy fence to keep yourself separate—not one of those little white picket fences that are just for decoration. They are easy to climb over, and you can see through them. At least in the beginning, make sure foods that are too tempting are out of sight and out of reach.

10) Test temptation

One of the secrets of skill building is finding the right amount of challenge so that you build confidence and avoid frustration. When you give yourself a chance to practice the skill of resisting small temptations, you are well on the road to avoiding temptation altogether.

Here's how one of the readers of my blog practiced testing temptation: *"I used to have a bad habit of constantly nibbling from the dish of candy at the office. I was usually the one who refilled the dish, and I usually put in Hershey Kisses, which I love. When I stopped restocking the dish, it was sometimes empty, but occasionally someone else refilled it. I decided to fill it with peppermint patties. I don't hate peppermint patties, but I'm not a big fan. I practiced walking past the dish over and over asking myself, 'Do I want a mint?' and answering 'No, I don't think so.'*

That was months ago. Now the peppermint patties are mostly absent, and so is my desire for the candy. No matter what's in the dish, M&Ms, peanut butter cups, or even my favorite, gold-wrapped almond kisses—99% of the time I can say, 'No, I don't think so' without even a twinge. Sometimes, I will have one, but only when I really want it, and I make a point of enjoying it thoroughly."

One of the best ways to do this is to practice saying "no" in a controlled environment. In the next chapter, I'll talk about the "when" skill of eating.

CHAPTER 2

*"Instead of trying to lose weight
while our body is in fat-storage mode,
we have to retrain our body to use fat
by shifting it into fat-releasing mode."*

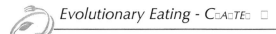

The Problem

We Try to Lose Weight
When We Need to Use Fat

In this chapter, I'm going to talk a lot about the term "weight loss." When you begin to learn how your body really works, you come to understand that the term "weight loss" is really a misnomer. It doesn't make sense. In fact, it can be really harmful to believe that we "lose weight." Let me explain.

Weight-loss myths

The real truth about weight loss is that there is no such thing. It's impossible to "lose weight." Your weight isn't like a backpack—it's not something you can carry around and then walk away from whenever you want.

Just think about it. How can you "lose" weight? Where does it go? Do we just misplace it? Of course not. We grow, but we don't really shrink. We can gain weight by either growing up or growing out (fat storage). It's convenient to think of "lose" as the opposite of "gain," but this isn't how the human body actually functions—our bodies never "lose weight."

What actually happens is we "use weight." When we gain more than we use, we get visibly bigger, and when we use more than we gain, the numbers on the scale will go down. Optimally, adults should be in balance or homeostasis—that's how we keep our weight stable over a lifetime. Up until the last 40 or 50 years, humans were able to manage this easily, even when food supply was variable.

But it gets more confusing. The term "lose weight" is actually incorrect in a second way. It's not just the word "lose" that's problematic—it's also the word "weight." Our body weight is actually composed of skin, skeleton, muscles, organs, vessels, nerves, fluids, and fat. Most of us are only interested in "losing" fat, not in losing "weight."

Animals use fat stores as a fuel reservoir. Human beings have one body, but it is composed of trillions of microscopic cells. These cells need a constant supply of fuel or they'll die, but we don't need to eat around the clock because we can store fuel in our bodies.

Contrast this with breathing. Cells also need oxygen or they will die. We have no way of "storing oxygen," so we must breathe air continuously. We breathe in air, and our respiratory system extracts the oxygen required by the cells. We eat food, and our digestive system extracts the fuel and chemical nutrients required by the cells. What can't be used right away can be stored for later in the form of fat.

Fat is stored "geographically" all over the body, but it is contained in special cells called adipocytes (fat cells). Collectively, fat is called adipose tissue. We tend to think of our fat as something lumped onto our bodies like frosting on cake, or butter on bread, but adipose tissue doesn't just contain fat—it hormonally controls it. It's crucial for us to understand the difference because you can't use fat for fuel unless it is released—and that means getting hormones working for you instead of against you. (Don't worry, you're going to learn how!)

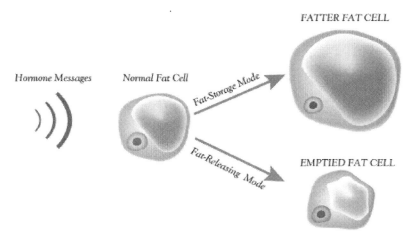

Fat cells "decide" to store more fat for the future or to release fat to be used for energy in response to hormonal signals.

When the body is functioning well, with adequate food in the environment and some reserve fuel in the fat stores, the adipose tissue allows individual fat cells to release the fat globule to be used as fuel for the cells. Starvation is what happens when there is no food in the environment, and no fat globules in the fat cells. That's when you really "lose weight" because the body will begin digesting itself—muscle tissue, organs, etc. are used as fuel.

Remember, cells must always have fuel, or they will die. In starvation, muscles will shrivel and organs can even wither because the body knows that these can "grow back" when food becomes available again. So the body doesn't store building blocks, it only stores fuel. When food is available in the environment, the size and weight of our organs, skin, skeleton, and blood volume remain relatively stable.

Because of the hormone testosterone, males can increase their muscle mass. But muscles are like tiny leaky balloons. In order to stay "plumped up," they have to be continuously "pumped up" with effort, extra protein, and a hormonally favorable environment; otherwise, they deflate back to their relatively flat default state.

Fat doesn't work that way. It is happy to "plump up" when there is extra fuel. Under the right hormonal conditions (probably the ones in your body right now), these fat cells become hoarders that hold on to their fat globule, and even add to it.

Our bodies will only use our weight when we are in a state of starvation. When your fat stores are depleted, your body starts to use your muscle mass for fuel. That, of course, is not our goal. When everything is working the way it should be, our bodies are continually using fat as a fuel source, making it quite easy to maintain a natural, healthy weight.

Through dieting, calorie restricting, and other weight-loss methods, however, this weight-regulating mechanism often becomes dysfunctional. What happens hormonally is that our bodies shift from a state called "fat-releasing mode" into a perpetual and chronic state of "fat-storage mode."

If you are struggling with your weight, or if you have ever dieted in the past, it's likely that your body is stuck in the state of fat-storage mode.

But don't worry; you're not broken! Your body is simply confused. We just need to re-train it to use your fat stores as a fuel source instead of storing all the food you eat as fat.

Fat-releasing mode and fat-storage mode

Each and every one of us has a weight-regulating mechanism that determines how much fat our bodies release and store. Because many factors influence our weight-regulating mechanism, it is not something that can be changed easily.

In a normal functioning individual, the weight-regulating mechanism shifts our hormonal status between fat-storage mode and fat-releasing mode throughout the day. For simplicity, we can say that when we eat, we use a small amount of that food for immediate energy needs, and the rest is sent to the fat stores for storage. When we are not eating, fat is released from the fat stores so it can be used as fuel.

Here is this process in its simplest form.
- When we eat, our bodies shift into fat-storage mode.
- When we stop eating, our bodies shift into fat-releasing mode.

When you try to "lose weight" too quickly, or when you restrict calories for a long period of time, you disrupt your weight-regulating mechanism.

Our bodies are designed to shift from a balance of fat storing/fat releasing (healthy homeostasis) to a chronic state of fat storing. Fat-storage mode is actually a safety mechanism. When our body begins receiving information that there is less food in the environment (which happens with dieting and weight-loss programs), it is designed to store and hoard as many calories as it can from any food that you eat.

As I said earlier, humans are the naturally fattest species on Earth. We have ten times the number of fat cells expected for mammals of our size. Why? The quick answer is that humans differ from the other animals most dramatically because of our large brain — it's four times bigger than that of our "brainy cousin," the chimpanzee. Leopards have spots and humans have thoughts — it's what distinguishes us in the animal kingdom.

Our big brain is a fuel guzzler. Although it is only 2% of our "weight," it uses 20 to 25 percent of the fuel—24 hours a day—whether we are thinking, sleeping, or running around.

Evolution didn't just give humans big brains; it also provided an insurance policy, a very different fat-storage system to protect it. It is a mechanism that served us well when there was actual food scarcity.

But in a world of food abundance, we no longer need to be constantly storing fat. We now have the technology to store food in our pantries rather than our bottoms; we just have to re-train our brain so that it understands this process.

Our fat stores are interested in the future—the future in terms of food supply, and also the future in terms of the next generation. We have known for a long time that fat and fertility go hand in hand. Ancient artwork proves it (Google "Venus of Willendorf," for one example).

So the bad news for your butt is that humans are fat—and the worse news for your butt is that female humans are even fatter (which is why female hormones make your butt fat). This is nature's way of giving an "extra insurance policy" for the bun in oven—because that bun will have its own brain. In short, women go into fat-storage mode more easily, and cling to it longer and harder than men.

This isn't news to any woman who started a diet with her husband or boyfriend; he is much more likely to get results faster. That's why so many women experience the same painful, frustrating situation—they are trying to shed unwanted fat while their bodies are in fat-storage mode.

Even though the modern environment is one of perpetual food abundance, physiologically, and hormonally, chronic dieting alerts the body to a long winter of food scarcity ahead. Until very recently, humans lived in a variety of climates, but all experienced the same food environment and cycle. This cycle was either scarcity-abundance-scarcity or famine-feast-famine.

We have many safeguards in place to make sure we gorge and store during feast times. We fatten up our body pantries because famine (winter) will surely be coming, and there will be no food.

Though we can live without food, we cannot live without fuel. Those fat stores are the lifeline that sustains us until food becomes available and the cycle begins again. Most animals give birth in springtime when the food begins to return.

Mammals, including humans, must grow their young inside their bodies. Women really are "eating for two," but in the natural world they must eat for two even before pregnancy because humans (like other mammals) are traditionally pregnant during the winter—the time of traditional food scarcity.

That's what makes females different. All humans are designed for individual survival, but females have special modifications to ensure species survival. Female hormones have a tremendous impact on many aspects of physiology—not only the physical fat stores, but also motivation and behavior. This is why females have so many more food "issues," like eating disorders, binging, cravings, and tendencies to become overweight or obese.

Women's wiring and chemicals create more intense temptation, and more difficulty resisting it. Many adult women in the modern world struggle constantly with their weight because their bodies are running in a chronic state of fat-storage mode, which means that everything they eat is prioritized in terms of storage rather than usage.

And what happens then? These women feel terrible because they can't "lose" weight, so they go on another "weight loss" program!!! This does nothing except make the problem much, much worse.

If you are in fat-storage mode, it doesn't matter how little you eat, or how much exercise you do. In fat-storage mode it will be extremely difficult to release any fat from your body.

Anything you eat will be sent straight to the fat stores, and those same fat stores will try to hoard as much of that energy as possible. An apt analogy is that when you're in fat-storage

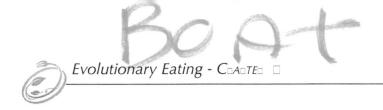

mode, it's like being in a boat that has been inadequately prepared for sea. It hasn't been sealed correctly (prepared for the "water environment"), and has lots of leaks in it.

These leaks were invisible when the boat was on dry land (the old food environment), but once you set sail, water starts to seep in from this place, then that place, and soon from all over the place. That's the modern food environment—lots of food assaulting you from all over.

As the water comes in, you are trying to bail it out as fast as possible (dieting and exercise), but it doesn't matter how hard you try because the water keeps filling up the boat faster than you are able to bail it (as your body stores and hoards quicker and more effectively than you can "lose" it). Over time, even the bucket can develop leaks (the diet and exercise don't work as well). Now you have to work twice as hard just to keep up. What a nightmare!

This is where we are with dieting. It doesn't matter how much we think we can "lose," as our body can also accumulate and store fat quicker than we are able to lose it.

So, instead of trying to lose weight while our body is in fat-storage mode, we have to retrain our body to use fat by shifting it into fat-releasing mode. Instead of bailing all the water that is coming from the leaks, we need to fix the underlying problem.

We need to fix the leaks. We need to make our boats, or rather our bodies, "seaworthy." And we do that by making our hormones work for us rather than against us.

This principle is so important. We've all been focusing on bailing the water instead of properly preparing our bodies to sail the seas of the modern world. When we're overly and unattractively fat, the problem is that we have leaks in our behavior. Leaks in our behavior create hormonal imbalances in our bodies.

The end results are a constant state of fat accumulation, no matter how much we sweat from exercise, or suffer from hunger and food preoccupation. So please stop this dieting and weight-loss madness. Not only does it not work, but it makes matters worse. It creates more leaks in our boat.

We have to stop trying to lose weight, and instead learn how to use fat. We have to shift our body's internal status from fat-storage mode back into fat-releasing mode. We do this by plugging the leaks in our behavior. These behaviors are the fundamental skills of eating.

The Solution

Learn the "When" Skill of Eating

Wouldn't it be nice if we really could melt away the fat just by increasing the "burn?" Unfortunately, this is magical or infomercial thinking. If you are going to persist in thinking of your fat as a lump of Crisco, then let's at least complete the image—to melt the Crisco, you have to open the can. You have to release the fat.

Let's continue with our leaky-boat analogy. Here's the worst-case scenario: you are adrift at sea (lost in the food court at the mall, the enticing smell of Cinnabons in the air). There is no hope in sight. (They are actually giving away "free samples.") There is water coming in from multiple "invisible leaks"—many external cues to eat NOW!

You're getting nowhere with your fat-loss plan because you can't paddle when you're bailing water. You have been trying many buckets (diet and exercise plans), and are currently using a discarded Starbucks Grande skinny-latte cup. In other words, you are eating 800 calories a day and arrived at the food court after your morning run… Translation: you are ravenously hungry and the skinny latte isn't cutting it.

Exhausted and stressed, you decide to "indulge" this once, and have a big low-fat bran muffin. This is basically the same as "stopping your bailing to rest for just a minute." It really doesn't satisfy you, plus you figure that since you've now broken your diet, you might as well take a break for the day and start again tomorrow.

After a day of nibbling on sweet treats, and maybe even a binge (it's hard to control your appetite once it gets loose), you fall asleep after a glass of wine—or three—and wake up to find that your scale has defied the laws of physics—you have gained several "pounds," even though you didn't eat tens of thousands of calories.

This is the same as having taken a nap in your boat and awakening to find the water level inside has risen to an alarming level. You are now in imminent danger of going under—maybe permanently. You immediately pick up the Starbucks cup and start bailing as fast as you can, all the while frantically scanning your choppy water for help in the form of a better bucket (diet and/or exercise program/trainer, or some other desperate measure).

Sound familiar? Of course it does. Did you think you were alone? No, this is common—horribly and tragically common.

You are out at sea, and not only is that diet not saving you, it's drowning you. You have to fix the boat.

You need to shift from fat-storage mode to fat-releasing mode. Otherwise, any time...any time...you take a break, you will take on extra water (extra weight) that you will have to work two, three, or even ten times harder to get rid of.

And remember, all the while, you are busy bailing. You can't paddle. You can't get where you want to be.

There is a solution. It will take a bit of effort and persistence, but mostly it takes a lot of courage—courage to stop bailing.

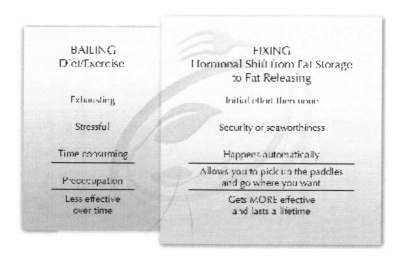

BAILING Diet/Exercise	FIXING Hormonal Shift from Fat Storage to Fat Releasing
Exhausting	Initial effort then none
Stressful	Security of seaworthiness
Time consuming	Happens automatically
Preoccupation	Allows you to pick up the paddles and go where you want
Less effective over time	Gets MORE effective and lasts a lifetime

94

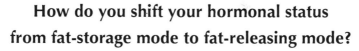

How do you shift your hormonal status from fat-storage mode to fat-releasing mode?

You use the right ingredients and apply the right techniques. You focus on the most important leaks first—the ones in the BOTTOM of the boat! They are the ones that are always taking on water.

The hormone we have to fix first is insulin, and the quickest, safest, and most effective way to fix insulin problems is by adjusting when you eat.

The wonderful bonus benefit is that these techniques don't just affect insulin, but also have an effect on other weight-regulating hormones. There are many hormones in the body, and they all interact with each other rather than working separately.

These hormones include insulin, leptin, and ghrelin. Neuro-chemicals, such as dopamine, serotonin, and Neuropeptide Y, also all affect your hormonal status, and what you need to change to shift your body into fat-releasing mode. Here, however, we are just going to explore one of the hormones—insulin.

Insulin is the storage hormone

I call insulin the "storage hormone" because its primary purpose is to store the food we eat somewhere in the body—in the liver, in the muscle cells; in the fat cells.

95

Wherever insulin thinks the fuel is needed, that's where it is going to store it. In the modern world, where food is abundant and we frequently graze and feast, insulin has the dirty, time-consuming job of shoving more fat into your already overstuffed fat cells.

There are trillions of cells in every human body. Each one of these cells requires energy to function and survive.

As you can imagine, with that many cells, there is quite a bit of competition for which gets the most energy. Which cells have priority? The brain cells? The muscle cells? What about the fat cells? An even better question may be: Who decides where the energy goes? The answer isn't really a "who," it's a "what." And that "what" is insulin.

Most people have heard about insulin—they know it regulates blood sugar in both normal people, and those with diabetes. Regulating blood sugar is important because high blood sugar, or hyperglycemia, is poisonous to cells, organs, and blood vessels.

The modern world has a lot of sugar and starch—things that make blood sugar go up. (I'll cover this further in the "What" eating skill chapter.) But in the natural world—the one in which humans evolved—the type and quantity of food that makes blood sugar go sky high was just not available.

So insulin's original role wasn't specifically blood-sugar management, but rather fuel management, in general.

The modern world is placing a huge burden on insulin, so it's no surprise that just like a person who is chronically overworked and under-appreciated, insulin is turning against us, either by open rebellion (the explosion of type 2 diabetes in adults, and even children), or by passive-aggressive resistance (people getting stuck in fat-storage mode, putting on fat no matter what we do).

When people are in fat-storage mode, or chronic insulin dominance, normal priorities get scrambled. All cells need fuel, but fuel doesn't get into the cells unless insulin opens the door. In fat-storage mode, many of our cells, like those in our muscles that need to move, become resistant to insulin.

Insulin knocks on the door announcing the fuel delivery, but the muscle cells pretend nobody is home. Instead, they just call the brain and tell it that no fuel was delivered, creating a whole new set of problems. Unlike muscle cells, however, fat cells are very easy-going; they don't really resist insulin.

When insulin comes knocking, the fat cells always open the door. But fat cells have another problem—when insulin is hanging around, they won't let the fat out! When the other cells need to make a withdrawal, the fat cells give them an infuriating "out of service" message.

There are many, many factors (all of which are studied in exquisite detail in pristine laboratory settings) that affect insulin secretion. Personally, I like a high-payoff approach to fixing things. Instead of trying to tackle all the problems at once, let's deal with the ones that will give you most bang for your buck.

The most important eating skill to master—the biggest bang—is also the first one we ever learn: when to eat. Before a baby is born, it doesn't need to eat. The mother provides oxygen, nutrients, and fuel for the cells of the growing baby. So for simplicity's sake, you could say a fetus eats "continuously." As soon as the baby is born, it must begin to breathe and eat to keep all those cells alive and happy.

Babies take their first cry, and then begin to breathe regularly and continuously. Babies take their first gulp, and start to eat intermittently. At first, they have to eat very frequently, but as digestive and hormonal systems mature, the baby can "wait" for longer and longer intervals. And that is what used to happen. Babies had "feedings," small children had frequent smaller meals, and larger children and grownups ate two or three times a day.

Right after we eat, there is fuel circulating in the blood stream. Insulin directs this fuel into cells for immediate use. Because a meal is going to contain extra fuel, the extra fuel has to be stored away safely, and retrieved later (assuming we actually have an interval between meals), when there is no longer fuel in the bloodstream. The main function of fat cells is to store this energy when we have a surplus, and then to release that energy for use when we have a deficit.

The only "problem" with this mechanism is that it only works well when we have regular eating intervals; when there is insulin circulating in our bloodstream, we are in "fat-storing" mode, and when there is little or no insulin, we are in "fat-releasing" mode. When you constantly eat, your levels of insulin remain high, and thus most of the food you eat gets stored instead of used for your basic energy needs.

This can set up a scenario in which you are eating lots and lots of food, but the energy from that food is being shunted into your fat cells via insulin, while all of your other cells are hungry. Basically, you are starving while getting fat.

This process was summed up by Gary Taubes, author of the fantastic books, *Good Calories, Bad Calories* and *Why We Get Fat,* when he said, "We don't get fat because we eat more; we eat more because we are getting fat."

In other words, when we are in fat-storage mode, our bodies crave more and more food. We really have no choice but to continue eating because the food that we eat goes primarily into fat storage, and only a small amount gets used for our immediate energy needs. As most dieters can attest, it really is a nightmare situation.

If insulin is the problem, then snacking is the cause

Although insulin is the storage hormone, it is not the enemy. We need insulin because it performs a vital job within our bodies. But what we need to understand is that although we need insulin, we don't need it all the time.

To create a healthy balance, there need to be times when we are not eating. When we are "fasting," which is what happens "between meals" (that's why the first meal of the day is called "breakfast"), there is little or no insulin in our bloodstream. During this time, therefore, our body's balance shifts towards fat-releasing mode.

When insulin isn't hoarding it, the fat can be released to act as a fuel source when we are not eating. This is what it means to use fat. Generally, this process occurs naturally, but a behavior has emerged in the past 40 years that has completely disrupted this mechanism. That behavior is called snacking.

At no time in human history has snacking been a normal behavior. Humans are not grazing animals. Our digestive and endocrine (hormone) systems are designed to have food-free intervals. We are designed to eat a meal, stop eating, and eat another meal sometime in the future.

The change from becoming meal eaters to snackers has had a lot to do with our environment. Our hormones and digestion might work best with intervals, but our brain and nervous system are optimized to be highly motivated to seek out and eat food when it is available. That was the only way for our species to survive and thrive.

Until recently, snacking wasn't really an option. Food was relatively scarce, and often required preparation before eating. In today's environment, there are 24/7s on every street corner, vending machines in every building, and pantries that can store many years' worth of food.

Our brains signal us to eat, and our culture no longer restrains us; it is socially acceptable to eat anytime and anywhere.

The combination of abundant food and no social boundaries means that many of us are eating all the time.

Humans have been around for millions of years, but even 100 years ago, we did not have the refrigeration, processing, or freeze-packaging technology to keep food edible. But just because we invented ways of preserving food doesn't mean that our genes mutated overnight.

Agriculture is hard labor. Farmers, who were the majority of people in the United States until the 1950s, would have to plant, grow, dig up, gather, and prepare the food, all before they were able to take a bite.

Today, we barely have to leave the sofa. For those who don't want to make even that much effort, there are super-sized bags of snack food on which we mindlessly munch while watching the television.

The data are clear—whether you're speaking about America, or anywhere else in the world, the single most important predictor of weight gain isn't how much you eat, but how OFTEN you eat.

Some of the most fat-resistant cultures are also the most culturally snack-resistant. The French don't even have a word for snack—they call it "le snack." In fact, they have a government-mandated anti-snacking culture that they resurrect when their toddlers start to get tubby. Called *puericulture,* the movement has been utilized in the past with great success, and is regaining popularity once again.

Basically it means no snacks, no second helpings, and supervised social mealtimes. It's intended for children, but since we all seem to eat like babies these days—on demand, wherever we are, using minimal utensils, without fuss or chewing required—perhaps we should take note of a movement with a history of success.

Instead, we devote billions of dollars, and buckets of sweat and tears, to the diet-and-fitness industry, and are happy with results that would make even a cancer doctor cringe. The chances of losing weight and keeping it off for more than two years is somewhere between one and four percent.

How would you feel if your doctor told you those were your odds of beating your cancer? The first thing we would do is get a second opinion—preferably from a doctor with a much higher success rate!

One of the common traits of skillful, competent eaters is that they all eat meals, and very few eat snacks. Many fitness professionals will tell you to eat six small meals a day. Well, that is good for business. I'm not in the fitness business, so I'm going to say point blank that snacks should never be a part of the human diet because there is no such thing as a healthy snack.

Snacking, as a behavior, is one of the biggest leaks we need to plug if we are going to regain control of our weight-regulating mechanism, and finally shift ourselves back from fat-storage into fat-releasing mode.

When you eat food, and sometimes when you even see or smell food, your body will secrete insulin, which is going to push you towards fat-storage mode. When you eat frequently, you will always have insulin circulating around, causing all the cells but fat cells to become insulin resistant.

Insulin also keeps you in fat storage because insulin blocks the adipocytes from releasing fat when it is needed for fuel. Eventually your fat cells get inflamed, sick, and dysfunctional—and so do you.

This doesn't happen at the same rate in all individuals— some people are genetically predisposed to become insulin resistant more easily.

The solution is simple. It may not be easy, but it is very simple:

- Eat two or three meals daily.
- Preferably on a regular schedule.
- And don't eat at any other times.

Learning the first skill of eating: WHEN to eat

When you are building skills, you are trying to change your habits. Keep your focus on behaviors, rather than results.

The first skill of *Evolutionary Eating* is learning when to eat. There are certain behaviors that you can learn and practice that will make you an adept "When" eater. Some of these behaviors are outlined in the quick-start strategies section of this chapter.

However, there is one behavior I insist almost everybody implement as soon as she or he can. That behavior is to eat meals only, and to cut out snacking entirely. It's okay to eat snack foods as long as they are a part of a meal. It is the behavior of snacking that is the major problem.

When you snack or eat between meals, your insulin hangs around for too long. This keeps your body in fat-storage mode. The most important first step is to restore normal insulin balance. Every time you eat (with a few exceptions,) insulin comes out. It has to be used up—it doesn't just "go away."

That means you must have food-free intervals because when people are in fat-storage mode they are insulin resistant, and it takes longer to get insulin back to zero. Unless your insulin is at zero, you are not releasing fat. If you are not releasing fat, then you can't use it. If you snack, you are stuck. Stop snacking.

P.S.: That means apples, apple pie, apple juice, and Apple Jacks cereal. That means any food or drink that has calories. In short, in the *Evolutionary Eating* mindset, snack (the bad kind) is a verb, not a noun. And the rule about snacking is a twist on a Nike slogan: Just DON'T do it.

The "WHEN" Skill of Eating

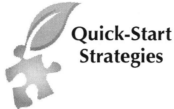

Quick-Start Strategies

1) Eat a real breakfast

Eating the right breakfast is important for people who need to re-regulate their leptin, an appetite-regulating hormone, but I also recommend eating breakfast for a different reason. Eating a good breakfast puts you in the right mindset, and it sets you up for the day. Having a real meal in the morning will give you the momentum to continue that mindset into the rest of the day.

If you grab something unsubstantial for breakfast, you almost give yourself permission to snack an hour or two later. That's not what you want. Breakfast doesn't have to be large, but it should be satisfying—be sure to include some fat and protein (as these foods have a lot more staying power).

2) Eat meals

Perhaps the single most important behavior for regulating your insulin is to eat meals. Using punctuation when they eat is a big step for many people.Start with easy sentences. Eat.

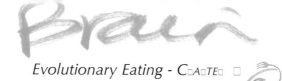
Stop. Eat. PERIOD. As you build skill, you can begin to handle all the fancy stuff, like semicolons and dashes. For now, you need to stick to well-defined basics. Start eating a meal. Finish eating a meal. Don't eat again until the next meal.

3) Be the boss of your brain

Your brain is in charge of motivating you to eat. In other words, hunger comes from your brain, not your belly. If you don't want your brain to bother you between meals, you must refrain from eating until the next meal.

Teach your brain that you mean business! Say to yourself, "I don't have to eat now. I can wait until dinner (or lunch or breakfast)." The more you practice not giving in to the snack attack, the less your brain will bug you and beg you.

4) Eat no more than three meals a day

With very few exceptions, there is no reason to eat between meals, or eat more than three meals a day. You are not a baby or a puppy.

If you take insulin or diabetes medication, you need to follow the advice of your physician. If you are healthy enough to go on "a diet," you are probably healthy enough to eat like an adult. Eat enough at one meal to last until the next. This is called satiety.

5) Eat regular meals

Insulin is just one of the many hormones that regulate your

hunger and appetite. Another hormone, called ghrelin, helps alert the brain that it might be time to eat.

To make ghrelin a helper instead of a hindrance, start off by eating regular meals on a schedule. That helps prevent ghrelin from bothering your brain all day long with distracting questions like "Would you like something to eat?" "How about just a bite?" and "Remember that pint of Cherry Garcia in the freezer?" For a quick start, eat regularly scheduled meals.

6) Plan meals

If you are like most chronic dieters, you have probably dabbled in "skipping meals" as a way of cutting calories. The problem is that your brain absolutely hates the prospect of not eating. Like a small child, however, your brain can be mollified with just a tiny bit of trickery—the addition of the simple word, "yet."

Never tell yourself you are "not eating." Always say that you are eating—you're just "not eating yet." On the other hand, you must then feed yourself when it is mealtime, or else your brain will know you're a big, fat liar, and turn on you, making you preoccupied with eating all of your waking hours (except for when it checks out while you are actually eating).

7) Eliminate nibbling!

We've mentioned that you need to stop snacking, but that

also includes nibbling, grazing, and any other variation of eating between meals. Mindless eating behavior is a surefire way to keep you in perpetual fat-storage mode.

What's worse is that when we snack and nibble, we often do so thoughtlessly. By the end of the day, we've completely forgotten that we have snacked at all!

We then give ourselves permission to overindulge at dinner time because we think, "I haven't eaten a thing all day!" The easiest way to stop this self-deception is just to eliminate nibbling altogether. Not only will it bring your levels of insulin down, but it will also allow you to monitor the amount you actually eat.

8) Establish a routine

As you are going to be eating regular meals, it is imperative that you establish a routine.

Because food holds such high survival value, your brain is constantly evaluating where your next meal is coming from. The brain loves habits and routines, especially when it comes to food. When you eat with a scheduled routine, your brain learns to expect food at certain times, which in turn tremendously decreases food preoccupation. This happens for a number of reasons, but primarily because your hunger hormones only get released when it is time to eat. (See "growlin' ghrelin" above and in the Prologue.) Reassure your brain that food is available by always eating at the same times, and your cravings will decrease greatly.

9) Learn to be comfortable with a little hunger

Most people do not quite understand hunger. Because hunger can sometimes be a little uncomfortable, we think it is an action signal: "Whenever I'm hungry, I must eat." The truth is that hunger a reminder that you should eat sometime in the future, not an action signal to eat immediately.

If you are eating meals, there may be brief periods of time when you feel a little hungry. A hunger pang is a hunger pain (and, like pain, it comes from your brain). You don't need to respond to a skinned knee like it's a compound fracture, and you don't have to respond to a rumbly tummy at 4 p.m. like all the food on Earth is going to vanish before dinnertime. If you wait instead of snacking, that hunger signal will subside. Remember, not yet.

10) Stop exaggerating

Words make worlds. Things you say out loud, especially things you say to other people, impact your thought processes. You are not starving, so don't make life even harder by saying it. Children are fond of announcing that if they don't have something to eat immediately, they will "starve to death." Answer your inner child with the wisdom of your inner granny: "You won't die before dinner. I promise."

11) Keep a "nibble notepad"

This is a little tip to help you "catch yourself" in the act of snacking.

Because we often nibble on food without even realizing it, it can be important in the beginning to keep a little notepad with you to write down all the bites that you take throughout the day. It's only at the end of the day when you look at your journal that you realize how much you've eaten!

Many people who nibble a lot will actually tell you that they don't, and they will believe it! So keep a little notepad close by, at least in the beginning. That's usually all it takes to become aware of your nibbling habits!

12) Technology to the rescue

Technology has given us many potentially fattening inventions, from microwaves to moving sidewalks. After all, that's what technology is—tools to make our lives easier.

So if a nibble notebook is a little too old school for you, develop the practice of taking a snapshot of anything you eat, especially nibbles. Make a point to review it daily, or better yet, send it to a friend (or an enemy) to hold yourself accountable.

13) Forget about "healthy" snacks

A lot of people understand that they shouldn't be snacking, yet they still do it if they are eating "healthy" food!

The reality is that "healthy" is just as much about when you eat as it is about what you eat. If you are eating between meals, you are engaging in an unhealthy behavior, no matter what food you are eating.

When you snack, you are reinforcing behavior; regularly practiced behavior becomes habit. We want you to develop the lifetime healthy habit of eating at mealtimes. Always remember, there is no such thing as a healthy snack!

14) Be decisive

When you make a decision about snacking, it needs to be definitive; either you are going to snack or you are not.

When you make a decision, your brain is less likely to fight with you. Here is why this is so important. If your brain thinks you will give in to its demands of snacking and nibbling, it will use energy to get you to do so.

It costs calories to argue with yourself, but it is worth it if your brain can get you to snack, resulting in a surplus of calories. This all reverts back to food preoccupation.

If you are stuck in a mode of thinking about snacking, you will eventually snack. If, on the other hand, you make a clear decision not to snack, then you have nothing to think about, and your brain won't constantly bug you with thoughts of eating.

15) No-No-No to nighttime eating

One of the most common snack times is evening. Eating in the four hours before bedtime creates tremendous problems with leptin, an appetite-regulating hormone. Unfortunately this is when most adults, especially women, have the strongest urge to eat.

This urge is so strong that I like to call it the "Zombie apocalypse" because it will turn some people in mindless, ravenous, food Zombies. If you tend to snack at night, get the food out of the house, find something else to occupy your mind, or try improving your sleep routine by getting to bed earlier.

16) Reward good behavior

One of the most common excuses used to justify snacking is that we deserve a little reward. It's like the old McDonald's slogan, "You deserve a break today." Don't make the mistake of substituting a punishment for a reward. Every single time you say NO to an impulsive urge to nosh or nibble, celebrate your little victory.

We spend a lot of time beating up on ourselves. When you reinforce good behavior, though, it is more likely to happen again. When you find yourself slipping into old habits, don't bother punishing yourself—it doesn't work. Instead, think of what you might do in the future when tempted in a similar manner. Write down your tips in your nibble notebook.

17) A final note—you don't need to carry a snack because you always have one with you!

We carry around a quick energy snack in our liver and our muscle cells. This snack is called glycogen, and it is a long chain of sugar. It's the emergency fuel supply—it's there to give us the burst of energy we need to avoid being eaten by a saber-toothed tiger. Unless we engage in some heavy-duty exercise, or fast for 10 to 12 hours, we always have a snack in the form of glycogen.

So you don't need to eat a snack for quick energy! Until your glycogen stores are depleted (including the sugar from your most recent meal or snack), your fat cells won't release fat to be used as fuel. When we snack, we are topping off our glycogen stores, and never allow our bodies any access to our fat stores. We stay stuck in fat-storage mode.

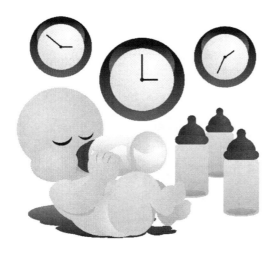

"Eating every few hours is for babies."

114

CHAPTER 3

*"For most of our history, we needed
to seek food, now we need to select it.
Modern humans must learn to
differentiate between real food and
things that appear to be food—
the food forgeries."*

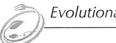

The Problem

We Count Calories
Instead of Counting Chemicals

While the first behavioral change I've addressed is "When," the "What," is also crucial. Infants don't have much choice over the "What" that they consume. All baby mammals are univores; they consume only one food—milk. No skill required! Mammals typically drink mother's milk until they are mature enough to obtain food on their own. Humans are the only mammals that have a true childhood. Because learning how to eat is such an important and complex skill, it takes many years for humans to become independent eaters.

Ironically, in the modern world many humans resume their defaults position of infancy, and are unable to feed themselves without the assistance of invisible adults—the food industry. The reality is that modern humans aren't terribly proficient in the skill of eating. This is why it is so easy to fool us with food forgeries.

Food forgeries look, feel, smell, and taste like food, but once they are digested, they can cause problems in the body because they are confusing to the cells.

117

Remember that we eat food, but our cells do not. Our cells run on the fuel and nutrients that are absorbed after the food has been digested into very basic chemical compounds. The body must recognize and identify those compounds to handle them appropriately.

Nowadays, much of the "food" recognized by our senses (vision, touch, hearing, smell, and taste) doesn't match what ends up in our digestive tract. It's likely that food forgeries were born of necessity. It's no coincidence that the first food forgery is "formula." Formula is a forgery of human milk—a clever copy that works well as a substitute. They say necessity is the mother of invention, and this is a perfect example. What do you feed starving babies when there is no breast milk?

You feed them modified cow's milk or modified soy juice. You feed them so that they are not starving, and then you work on the food to make it as much like the original as possible. It will never be perfect, but over time we can make it better—a better "copy" (looks and taste like milk), and a more nourishing product (supplies the body with required chemicals). Formula may not be "as good as" mother's milk, but it is certainly better than nothing.

Another reason for food forgeries is economic. Real food is costly, often prohibitively. When people are starving, they will eat anything to make the pain of an empty belly go away. People will certainly eat food forgeries, especially when that is all they can afford.

During times of war, real food usually becomes scarce and expensive. Margarine, which is congealed oil chemically altered to resemble butter, is a perfect example. We "invented" margarine because real butter was either unavailable or terribly expensive. What was once done out of necessity is now done for profit.

Packaged food is always a food forgery — it mimics real food and costs less. Though it's true that it costs the consumer (us) less, we forget that a great deal of the savings, in fact, goes into the pockets of the food producers.

Manufacturers, of course, only make what we are willing to buy, so they are constantly modifying their products and marketing new products.

Right now, the food producers know we care about healthy eating, nutrition, and obesity. They know consumers are much more likely to purchase items with labels that say "low in fat," "low in calories," "heart healthy," and "fortified," or "enriched" with vitamins and minerals, so they manufacture and market their products with that in mind.

Real food is already good for your brain, heart, and health. Real food has vitamins and minerals your body needs in the right proportions; it doesn't need to be enriched or fortified because the nutrition hasn't been stripped away in an effort to make it cheaper or extend its shelf life.

There is so much to learn about the "What" that it is easy to just throw up your hands. So many sources are telling you so many things. But keep in mind that it has never been easy for humans to know what to eat. We have always had to struggle to find food that makes us healthy and satisfied.

Keep in mind that humans are still hunter-gatherers. The task of traditional hunter-gatherers was to seek; the task of modern hunter-gatherers is to select. We must learn to differentiate between real food and things that appear to be food — the food forgeries. Most animals are born with instinctive food knowledge. They have an inborn drive to eat a diet that is species-appropriate. Humans are different. We aren't born knowing what to eat; it is something we must learn. Even under the best of circumstances, this takes a long time.

How we learned about food for millions of years

We don't really think about eating as something we learn because it is one of those things that happen automatically when we observe other people. It's not like learning to drive; it's like learning to speak.

Humans start out univores (milk), but we become omnivores. Some people think omnivores can eat anything, but they are wrong — omnivores have a specific diet just like all other animals. All animals must eat food appropriate for their digestive system and specific needs.

Humans have a small digestive system and large brain. We evolved to use our brain to choose foods that give us the most brain benefit. For millions of years, we were tribal hunter-gathers. We roamed over a fairly large habitat, learning about what plant and animal products were safe and nourishing, or how to prepare them so they were safe, storable, and health enhancing. We learned by observing the behavior of family, friends, and community, absorbing the food culture that was appropriate to the environment where we lived and raised future generations.

How we learned about food for millions of minutes

That was how we learned about new and/or unfamiliar foods in the past. Today is a little different. In today's world, instead of considering foods in terms of the nourishment they provide for our brains and body, the number one factor we use to determine what to eat is something called calories. But we still learn about eating the same old way—we watch how the people around us eat. For the past 40 years, most of the women we watch have been on a new thing called "a diet."

Most diets involve counting and cutting calories. Under laboratory conditions, this might work, but clearly it doesn't work in real life. If it did, we wouldn't have thousands of diets; we would have one--and that one would actually work. Calories are "measured" by putting a dab of food in a dish and calculating how much fire it takes to burn it to ash.

The instrument, called a bomb calorimeter, can be used in a high school science class. Unfortunately, your body isn't a bomb calorimeter, yet we pay more attention that number than we ever did in science class (especially chemistry). Here's a good example:

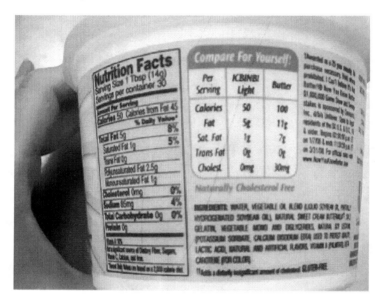

Counting calories when we read product labels has not made us slimmer.

We are missing out on a more important fact: all those ingredients are just FAKE ingredients, based on chemicals and health claims.

It doesn't take a statistician to show the relationship between dieting and weight. Dieting hasn't worked the way the scientists predicted, and we practiced. We dieted—we lost, we gained, and we got fat and fatter.

In the natural world, things that taste good and are edible, are usually food. Mother Nature has an organic restaurant for the planet Earth. Because humans weren't satisfied with the menu choices and meal times, though, we started to make our own food. We began with agriculture, our greatest technological feat.

Guess what wasn't on mother nature's menu? Bread.

There are fruits and vegetables in nature—there are even grains, which are grass seeds. Humans probably would have died out as a species if we hadn't discovered a way to coax these foodstuffs from the earth. We also started to raise animals for the food they could provide us. We fed them, and they fed us with their eggs, milk, and meat.

For 10,000 years, we've changed the menu at Mother Earth's country cafe by offering selections that weren't necessarily seasonal or abundant. The Earth doesn't make gardens or amber fields of grain—people do. These foods kept us from starvation.

Guess what wasn't in mother nature's kitchen? Machines.

You could say that, for the past 10,000 years, we have "modified" food, but we really didn't start to manufacture it until about a century ago.

Machines allow us to manufacture food because we are able to mechanically and chemically alter it. Because it looks and tastes like food, we assume it's as good for us as real, natural food. And because we have long lifespans, we haven't had the opportunity to see what consuming such "food" can do to a species over time.

In the laboratory, we run experiments on mice and fruit flies because they reproduce quickly, and you observe what happens over lifespans and generations. We are part of a food (or more accurately "food forgeries") experiment, but because we don't have the lifespan of fruit flies, we're just beginning to see and understand the outcome of consuming these foods. And the results are not pretty.

Humans live a long time. We need those lives to be healthy. Otherwise, what is the point of them? We don't have the ability to study the future generations to determine why our health seems to be deteriorating. So it might be a good time to study the past.

Fossilized bones tell us that our ancient ancestors often died young, usually from accidents, food shortages, or infectious disease. If they escaped these perils, they frequently enjoyed excellent health into their later years. They had no medical bills, but apparently they also had far fewer medical problems. They were sometimes skinny and sometimes starving, but they were rarely fat, even when they lived where food was plentiful.

Humans managed to survive and often thrive without knowledge of calories or nutrition. There was no need to label food as organic because there was no other kind of food. We had no need to distinguish food from food forgeries.

We evolved into the most adaptable species on earth—we can survive in any environment, including the modern one. But we can't expect to thrive on poor food forgeries.

Guess who wasn't on mother nature's payroll? Marketers.

Marketing is applied psychology. Marketers understand how to grab our attention and direct our purchases in a way that benefits their clients (and we are not their clients).

Marketers know we care about our health, and the health of our families. They also know we care a lot about value—we don't want to pay too much. It's predictable human nature that if we think two things are equivalent, we will choose the one that costs less, or gives us more for the same money.

Humans tend to care more about the short term, and have a hard time processing decisions that only affect us in the future. We get "fuzzy" when bombarded with numbers and expert opinions. We look for shortcuts and simplicity—that is just our nature. We also care a lot about our looks, especially if we are female. We don't want to be fat.

Women in particular will do anything that experts or the numbers or the marketers tell them will help them be thin — as long as isn't too complicated, expensive, or difficult.

Below is a chart of the things we would like to care about, but don't because our brains like things to be simple, effortless, and immediately gratifying.

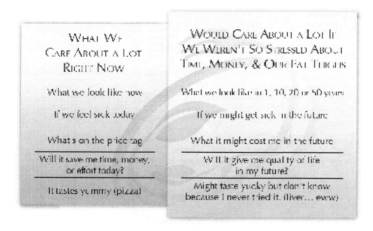

What We Care About a Lot Right Now	Would Care About a Lot If We Weren't So Stressed About Time, Money, & Our Fat Thighs
What we look like now	What we look like in 1, 10, 20 or 50 years
If we feel sick today	If we might get sick in the future
What's on the price tag	What it might cost me in the future
Will it save me time, money, or effort today?	Will it give me quality of life in my future?
It tastes yummy (pizza)	Might taste yucky but don't know because I never tried it. (liver... eww)

Real food provides nourishment (building blocks), sustenance (fuel), and celebration (social connectedness): all things that are important.

We must start to understand the difference between value and cost, or we will continue to pay a high price with our loss of wellness.

Calories and chemicals

Most people have lost the ability to distinguish between what is food, and what is not. We think that just because it is being sold in the supermarket, or the nearest 7-11, it must be food.

In truth, there are many things being sold as items that we can consume, but these items are "food-like" substances. They are not food at all. What good are calories if counting them has no benefits?

The people who know the most about calories are those that have been on the most diets. It seems that the more unsuccessful you are at weight maintenance, the more knowledge you will have about the calorie content of food. It makes perfect sense, since we know dieting doesn't work. Calorie counting is just another cog in the diet wheel.

Here is a quick and easy list to help you understand the difference between food and faux food, and the reasons you should fear chemicals instead of calories:

🪶 The items we eat in the modern world can be divided into two categories: food and forgeries.

🪶 Food is something that was once alive, either of plant or animal origin. (This includes fish.) It has no added ingredients. It has very little rubbish (chemicals/things our bodies cannot use). Before the advent of the food industry, this

127

type of food was what we always ate because that was all that was available to us. Food is the natural staple of a human diet.

Forgeries are copies of real food, things we can eat that are man-made. Non-food contains man-made chemicals and man-made preservatives, and it is created using man-made industrial machinery capable of extremely high temperatures and pressures.

These non-foods arrived when we started to take food in its natural form and change it into something different. Food producers can fool us into thinking that the copy is the same as the original because of the way they process, package, and market the forgeries.

When you go to the grocery store today, you will find that most of the "foods" are really just clever knockoffs of the real thing, often sold at a bargain price. Americans spend about 90% of their food dollars on processed food. For the first time in history, people are eating more non-food than they are food.

We pay attention to the calories because we have been told that is the only way to control our weight. We then turn a blind eye to the flaws of this low-calorie, low-cost "food," which has a vast number of chemicals added to it. We are exposed to thousands and thousands of new chemicals every year in the form of pesticides, preservatives, additives, artificial colors and flavor, and texture enhancements.

Eating non-foods is damaging to us for a whole lot of reasons, but it's a double blow that the food we are eating to try to get skinny is actually making us fatter—especially around our middles.

When we eat, some of our food isn't absorbed; it is eliminated as waste. But with so many chemicals on and in our food, we are absorbing a lot of "waste." (We can measure these chemicals in our blood, saliva, and hair.)

Waste inside of our body is a toxin—it can't be used or recycled into building blocks or fuel. Toxins are usually sent to the liver to be neutralized and then eliminated by the body.

Unfortunately, the liver can only deal with so much. If there are too many toxins in your body (which is always the case when you eat non-foods), the toxins are sent to the fat cells for storage.

Because toxins are dangerous, the body sends them into the fat cells so they will be isolated from the rest of the body. That way, they can be released at some later stage when the liver is not under such toxic pressure.

So a build-up of toxins from eating non-food is one of the main reasons that we get fat. But it's also one of the main reasons that we stay fat. If your body cannot deal with those toxins, it's going to keep them locked up in the fat cells. Your body won't release any fat because the fat is needed to protect your body from the toxins.

The toxics crowded into fat cells release loads of inflammatory chemicals that cause stubborn fat deposits, especially in the abdominal area. You can decrease your caloric intake, but your body will respond by guarding the fat at the expense of other tissues, and your metabolic rate. So you don't just lose your waistline, you lose your wellness.

This is the double-whammy you get from eating non-foods. They make you accumulate fat, and they make you hoard fat. They disrupt your weight-regulating mechanism; they keep insulin chronically high; they keep you in fat-storage mode; and they take you out of balance with many of your other hormones.

So the first step you need to take is to forget about calories. Not only are they irrelevant, but counting them can often be harmful because that often encourages you to consume a lot more non-food than you normally would.

The second step is to shift your attention from calories to food. You need to learn what food actually is, what food you should be eating, how to distinguish between real food and non-food, how to source real food, and what types of real food are important to eat. This is a skill—the skill of what to eat.

The third step is to learn about value. Forgeries are always cheaper than the real thing, but they don't and won't hold their value. If the things you value most are convenience, calories, and cost, you are in the same position of most modern Americans—but it doesn't have to be that way.

When you learn how to differentiate the food from the forgeries, and only pay for the real thing, you are investing in the most valuable piece of art you will ever own...yourself.

The Solution

Learn the "What" Skill of Eating

You might have noticed that the "What" skill chapter is the longest in the *Evolutionary Eating*. If the "When" skill is the most important, the "What" skill is a close second.

The "What" skill also takes the longest to learn, whether you are a child or an adult. It's probably easier, in fact, for children because they have no preconceived notions.

I might as well get the bad news out of the way. The reality is that there are very few shortcuts to the What skill of eating. This is not a skill you can ever take for granted.

We must always keep refining our knowledge because our food supply is always changing. But if you have solid foundational skills, you will be able to navigate the new territory more easily and skillfully. It helps to build a community where you can get help and information from like-minded individuals.

For most people, understanding what to eat is extremely confusing because there is so much conflicting information and so many viewpoints.

I'm not going to be dictating exactly what you should be eating. Instead, I'm giving you the tools you need to determine what to eat before you pop it into your mouth. (Babies will put anything in their mouths that attracts their attention. So do many adults—we call those things "free samples.")

The first and perhaps most useful tool for the "What" skill is "The Food Test." If the item passes The Food Test, that item is most likely real food and is safe to consume. A failure of the test indicates that you are about to eat a non-food item, probably a clever food forgery. Skillful shoppers aren't so easily suckered!

The characteristics of (real) food

It's much easier to spot the differences between real food and cheap knock-offs when you use The Real Food Test.

1) Real food was once alive—that is the very definition of food. Choose things that are as close to the living state as possible—either plant or animal. That means naturally colorful vegetables, fruits, and herbs. It means meat, fish, eggs, or full-fat dairy products, like butter, yogurt, and cheese. Understand that since food was once ALIVE, it is now DEAD. A big hint

133

that food is real is that it SPOILS. That's what happens to living things after they are no longer alive. I know it's gross, but it is a really important distinction.

2) Real food is not created in a lab and doesn't require a factory. An example of this is vegetable oil—including margarine, salad dressings, and most processed food that contains soybean oil.

"Vegetable oils" is a misnomer, since vegetables aren't "oily." To get oil from soybeans, corn, canola seeds, sunflowers, and safflowers, they must be subjected to extraordinarily high temperatures and pressures.

These products must then be treated with chemical solvents, filtered, and deodorized; otherwise, you would spot these "forgeries" in a second because they would look like sludge or Vaseline!

Vegetable oils are high in inflammatory omega-6 fats that are implicated in a wide variety of diseases, like cancer, heart disease, arthritis, and diabetes. Steer clear!

3) Real food often needs preparation. Wouldn't it be great if we had an internal "mom" voice that said, "Don't put that in your mouth—you don't know where it has been and who has touched it!" The more steps between the food in its natural state and the final product you put in your mouth, the more likely your food is "a forgery." Real food often needs a little preparation. The good news is that it already tastes good! The better news is that you know exactly who had their "hands in your food."

4) The only ingredients in real food are "food." We are often asked, "What should I look for on the label?" Real food often doesn't have one. When you eat food you make your-self, you know what went into it. When you buy prepared or packaged food, it's really wishful thinking.

5) Real food provides our body with building blocks and fuel with a minimal amount of rubbish. We only get one body and it must last us a lifetime. Every moment of our lives, our cells are busy making whatever we need for maintenance, repair, and our daily activities.

Cells can make many of those necessary compounds, but not all of them. We call these nutrients "essential," or building blocks, because we must get them from our diet. Our cells also need a constant supply of fuel or energy. Anything that our body cannot use as building blocks or fuel is rubbish. Essential building blocks are certain proteins, fats, and micronutrients, like vitamins and minerals.

I Can't Believe It's Not Butter is a popular brand of marga-rine, for instance — a forgery food. If we ever needed evidence of how little "what" skill we have, that is it.

Basically, the brand name is "I'm a Forgery, But Buy Me Anyway." Hopefully, with your new skills, when you put this food forgery on your veggies, you will say, "It's definitely not butter, and I can't believe it's not better!"

The Real-Food Test gives you a fantastic initial framework for deciding what it is you should and shouldn't be eating. A great way to start changing your eating habits, as the title of this chapter suggests, is to stop counting calories and to start counting chemicals. This is just another way of saying, "Learn to identify what is real food and what is non-food."

All non-food contains some type of chemical that disrupts our hormonal balance, puts us into fat-storage mode, and therefore keeps us perpetually fat. A way to count chemicals is to apply The Real-Food Test to any item. If the item passes the test, it is safe to eat. If it fails, then leave it on the shelf.

Keep in mind that real food often costs more because it is harder to grow or raise. It doesn't become freakishly large or productive; other animals, like insects, and rodents, compete for it (and we have to outsmart them rather than kill them); and because real food spoils quickly, it must be handled and purchased in a timely fashion or the farmer won't be able to make a living.

Eliminating as many of the non-foods from your diet as possible will transform your body from a fat hoarder to a fat releaser. That's how we change our bodies for a lifetime.

Just one final point. When I say "Eliminate non-food," I'm not saying you need to restrict and never eat certain types of food again. You're learning skills here, not having rules dictated to you. It is completely up to you what you decide to buy and eat. I'm only interested in helping you get information that is important to you and your family, whether you are a family of one, two, or ten. Make, source, and find food that is good for you, good for the planet, and ALSO delicious!

If you're going to make real changes, you need to be able to sustain those changes for a lifetime. You need to eat food that you enjoy, or you're not going to continue eating it.

And you need to be willing to invest in your good health by spending money on real food. Counting pennies, or even dollars, is a poor short-term strategy because the cheap knock-off food forgeries are forcing our bodies to store large deposits of inflamed toxic fat—especially around our middles.

The good news is when we tighten our belts by shifting more of our income into Real-Food choices; in the long term we'll be able to wear that tight belt proudly and comfortably.

The "WHAT" Skill of Eating

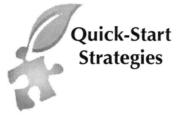

Quick-Start Strategies

1) Use the Real-Food Test

The Real-Food Test is a great quick-start strategy that you can use right away. It takes a little practice, but if you use the test, it won't be long before you are able to identify real foods and non-foods almost instantly.

If you're going to have any chance of getting your body into fat-releasing mode, this is something that you need to know and must do.

Why don't you start now? Open your fridge or pantry, grab an item, and run it through the Real-Food Test. I bet you'll be amazed at the results!

Americans spend 90% of their food dollars on processed food — most of which won't pass the Real-Food Test. So if most of your "foods" are "forgeries," you have a lot of company.

2) Dump the calorie counter

This is a huge challenge in the beginning of learning the skill of what to eat. For decades, many of us became convinced that calories were important. If you lived in a lab, that might be true, but just because data from lab rats give us important insights does not make us "lab rats."

"Calories-in, calories-out" is a poor strategy because it is too simplistic and too difficult. That's why the long-term outcome of this strategy is poor, especially if your body is in metabolic disarray from chronic dieting. I wouldn't tell you to just run faster if you had a sprained ankle, and I'm not going to tell you to just consume fewer calories if you are carrying excess body fat.

It will be hard to let go of a concept we have embraced so fanatically. But we must, because it hasn't just gotten us anywhere—it's gotten us worse than nowhere. It's gotten us to Fatland. When we didn't count calories, obesity was rare. The opposite is true today, despite posters, labels, and public-service announcements.

Ignoring calories may be difficult initially, but as you begin building your skills, you will see that learning what real food is, how to identify it, and how to avoid and eliminate the non-food items will serve you better in the long run.

3) Labels are just another way of marketing (selling)…

Food that has a label is often not food at all. Think of it as a forgery with a "sticker of authenticity." Food labels are not there to inform us; they are advertisements designed to make us buy. As a general rule, real foods do not have labels because they don't require them. A carrot is a carrot; we all know what it is. The same can be said for an egg, a tomato, or a piece of fish.

Non-foods have labels because (a) they contain more than one ingredient, some of which are not food at all, and (b) the label serves as a marketing tool to make us buy it. Without the label, we would most likely stick to real food, but with all the non-food health claims, such as "enriched," "fortified," "added vitamins," "healthy," etc., we get enticed into preferring, purchasing, and consuming them.

A simple strategy is to eat things that are recognizable and that have no label. This will cut out many non-food items from your diet.

4) Don't eat too many of the "right" foods

This is a common mistake that many people make, probably because of all the "Eat all you want and still lose weight" diets that are around today. It's easy to get our brains to accept the idea that eating "health food" makes you healthy, and eating more health food makes you even healthier. This is just wrong.

This misconception became popular because of the occurrence of vitamin deficiencies, ones that arise most commonly when someone (often the government or military) alters the food supply to make it less expensive.

When people become ill, those who altered the food figure out a "supplement" to prevent the disease, and add it back in. That's what enrichment is. It is a poor substitute for real food.

Pioneering nutritionist, Adele Davis, compared this to someone stealing 25 dollars from you and returning 99 cents. You are no longer broke; thus, you have been "enriched." That means with a little "nutrition" often comes much baggage — lots of unneeded fuel that will get stored as fat, and quite a bit of rubbish.

Many people consume huge amounts of food just because they think it is "nutrient rich," and will lead to better health.

A perfect example of this is orange juice. Many people gulp down a glass of this concentrated liquid daily. They don't consider that it takes several oranges to make a tiny glass, and a bag full for a large glass.

Who would eat a bag of oranges and then a full breakfast? But just one of those oranges would be a real food — packaged in the right proportions, and naturally full of vitamin C.

There would be no need to enrich with added synthetics (cheap, knock-off vitamins), or enhance for flavor. Ounce for ounce, orange juice has about the same amount of sugar as Coca-Cola. It doesn't have "better sugar." Sugar is sugar. The juice has a few more "nutrients" of dubious value, and it often has more preservatives.

Have an orange—it's real food, the "original" model for nutrition, and it's a lot more satisfying. Don't eat or drink more of something just because you think it is good for you. Just eat real food; it has everything that you need.

5) Don't be fooled by "low-fat" foods

Read this very carefully: *Eating foods that are high in fat does not make you fat. Eating foods low in fat does not make you thin.*

I've discussed the main fat-storing hormone, insulin. Insulin is usually released whenever we eat food, but not in the same amounts. Fat causes little or no insulin response, and protein stimulates a little more insulin, but at the same time stimulates other hormones that counteract it.

Carbohydrates (bread, pasta, cereal, rice, and sweet foods) are often low in fat, but because they increase blood sugar dramatically, they provoke the largest and most-sustained insulin response, especially when they are consumed without fat or protein. Low-fat foods have a lot of the fat taken out of them, but that fat is replaced by huge amounts of...sugar.

For example, man-made low-fat foods, such as low-fat yogurt, also contain large amounts of chemicals, which make them non-foods. So don't be fooled by the "low-fat" label; these non-foods put us into fat-storage mode, while their full-fat counterparts often don't! Also, we tend to eat a lot more "low-fat" food because we believe that since what we are eating is "low-fat," we can eat as much as we want without gaining weight!

6) Evoke the power of real-food substitution

You need to eat food that you enjoy, so elimination diets are a terrible long-term strategy. What we need to do instead is to substitute any non-food ingredients with real-food ingredients. So, if you're eating ice cream, the worst thing you can do is eat the "low- fat," chemical-laden, non-food version. Instead get the best quality, high-fat, organic ice cream.

Get it as close to its natural state as possible. An even better strategy is to make your own — it doesn't take that much time and you'll know exactly what's in it. Shouldn't a treat like ice cream take a little time and effort anyway?

Always try to substitute real food in and get non-food out. That's what will decrease your toxic load, and make your fat stores healthy, which in turn will set your hormonal status to "fat-releasing mode." Remember, if we have toxins locked in our fat cells, our body won't release the fat it doesn't need, so we'll stay stuck in fat-storage mode.

7) There's only one time you should eliminate real food

As long as you're eating real food, there are generally no other restrictions that you should make.

There is one exception, however. There are times when you may have one or two particular foods that you cannot stop eating. No matter what you do, you just can't stop thinking about this food. At times like these, you need an intervention — similar to a drug intervention.

Most people do not realize that food can be as addictive as any drug. If you can't stop obsessing over a particular food, you need to completely eliminate it from your life. You cannot eat foods like this in moderation; trying to do so is like asking a cocaine addict to moderate his intake. You must eliminate them.

It really is that serious. When you completely break the neural connection that this food has established in your brain, your craving will eventually subside. A common "real food" that has this quality is wheat.

8) Recoil from the oil

One of the most important aspects of *Evolutionary Eating* is learning about healthy and unhealthy fats. Your heart is a muscle, but your brain is basically a blob of fat. We need high-quality fat in our diets, but the fats most of us eat on a daily basis are highly processed substitutes that are also making our bodies inflamed, and are fat stores sticky. You can't burn the fat for fuel unless it is released from the fat cells.

You can determine what fats to avoid, and what fats to substitute, by following the Real-Food rules.

Never use vegetable oil, such as corn oil, cotton seed oil, soybean oil, or safflower oil. Also, understand that any manufactured product you buy will have these oils in them because they are cheaper and have a longer shelf life.

Almost all processed foods contain soybean oil because it's cheap, and improves texture and palatability.

Vegetable oils don't spoil like real food because they already became rancid during processing—the manufacturers just filtered, cleaned, and deodorized them so they look pretty in the bottle.

Safe oils in nature come from plants and animals that are naturally oily. They have been used in traditional cultures for thousands of years.

You can get oil from a coconut or an olive by mashing it with a rock. Try doing that with a corn kernel or a cottonseed!

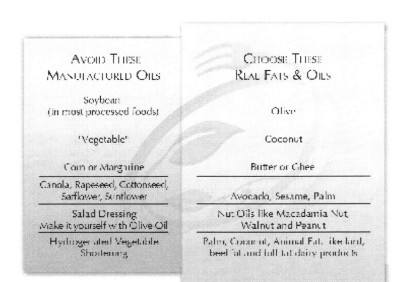

Avoid These Manufactured Oils	Choose These Real Fats & Oils
Soybean (in most processed foods)	Olive
"Vegetable"	Coconut
Corn or Margarine	Butter or Ghee
Canola, Rapeseed, Cottonseed, Safflower, Sunflower	Avocado, Sesame, Palm
Salad Dressing Make it yourself with Olive Oil	Nut Oils like Macadamia Nut, Walnut and Peanut
Hydrogenated Vegetable Shortening	Palm, Coconut, Animal Fat like lard, beef fat and full fat dairy products

9) Understand what you're putting in the frying pan

What's the difference between "fats" and "oils"? Fats are typically solid at room temperature because they are saturated. Your shirt is saturated when it holds as much water as it can and can't get any "wetter." A fat is saturated when it's holding as much hydrogen as it can and can't absorb any more chemicals. Saturated fats have gotten a bad rap—a very unwarranted bad rap.

The scientific literature is starting to trickle this information out, slowly and in a confusing manner. Scientific researchers are going to take their time about it because they were dead wrong about their earlier conclusions, and it cost many people health and happiness.

Saturated fats are safe as long as they are naturally saturated. The food producers manufactured saturated fats by taking manufactured, bad-for-you vegetable oils, and made them even worse by chemically exposing them to hydrogen and twisting them into a shape that was solid—that's what a bad-for-you "trans" fat is. Solid fats have a longer shelf life than oils (both the natural and unnatural varieties) because they can't pick up other "chemicals," like oxygen—they are already "saturated."

Cheaper hydrogenated vegetable oil "fats" are usually used in any processed or prepared (restaurants, take out) food that is fried. Why? Because it costs less. They aren't going to give you the more expensive variety when they can chemically alter it so our taste buds can't tell the difference (though our tummies can).

An important thing to remember about animal fats is that the best and healthiest fats come from animals eating a natural diet—and that usually means grass-fed and finished, or organic and pastured chickens and pigs.

10) Just because it has a "name" doesn't mean it's food

One of the many marketing ploys of the food industry is to give a food product composed of many ingredients a single name. LEGALLY (just in case you think laws always worked in your benefit), companies don't need to disclose "all the ingredients." That's a big problem with processed food.

So even when you think you know what went into a food product because of the ingredient list, you really don't.

Our brains tend to think of things with a name as single foods—but they're not. Sometimes we catch manufacturers on this. (Remember when they tried to pass off ketchup as food in school?) Most of the time, though, we won't notice, because that's how brains work—you can't pay attention to everything.

When you make your own food, it might have a lot of ingredients, but if all the ingredients are food, you still have "real food" with one name, which is not true for the processed equivalent. Check out the differences between an ingredient list (which is incomplete anyway) on a label and in a recipe for lasagna.

LABEL.	RECIPE

11) Beverages usually aren't real food, but they are lots of fuel

Nature doesn't make liquid food, except for milk. There is no "juice" in nature. There is water.

The average American consumes 156 pounds of sugar each year. More astounding, however, is that 35% of this sugar is consumed in liquid form.

When you drink this sugar, it bypasses your brain's satiety signals, which means it doesn't register as food—except in adding inches to your waistline. So, if you like to drink beverages other than water, try to stick to things that have a limited amount of sugar—tea, coffee, wine, and even milk is fine, as long as it is from grass-fed cows. It's not just the sugar that you are cutting out, of course; you're eliminating the chemicals that are in the man-made beverages.

12) Just because it contains a food word doesn't make it food

High fructose corn syrup (HFCS) is not corn, and fructose is not fruit. HFCS exemplifies the adage, "Be careful what you wish for."

We got what we asked for over and over again—cheap, tasty food. Though HFCS has only existed for a few decades, it's present in almost all processed, packaged, or prepared food. Because corn is subsidized (the government pays farmers to grow more corn than we need), it is very cheap.

A lot of this corn is fed to livestock, which makes meat very expensive. The remainder is processed into HFCS, which makes almost any food or drink taste more delicious, gives it a more attractive appearance, and prolongs its shelf life—all for less money than sugar from sugar cane (which is already inexpensive).

We are lapping it up and, as a result, we are losing our "laps." This cheap, ubiquitous non-food is causing our bellies to spill out over waistbands in a variety of unhealthy and unattractive bulges.

When you eat real food, it's easier to avoid this chemical. That's a good thing because fructose seems to be playing a role in many chronic illnesses, from high blood pressure to heart attacks. It puts a tremendous toxic burden on the liver—we are now finding children are developing fatty infiltration in their livers like alcoholics.

It's not just the booze that will kill you—modern beverages from soft drinks to sports drinks are loaded with this poisonous, "non-corn" food forgery.

13) Plan your shopping

A lot of weight gain can be limited by being conscious of the food you bring into your house. Much of our overeating, after all, is done at home. Keeping non-foods and your problem foods out of the house is a great start. Keeping real food in the house is also of great importance because it makes it much more likely that that is what you will eat. When you go food shopping, there are a few important rules you should consider.

The first is making a shopping list and sticking to it. When you make a shopping list, do it in a safe environment—your home. This means that you will reduce your susceptibility to the clever marketing techniques of supermarkets. Finally, don't go food shopping on an empty stomach!

Letting yourself get hungry is okay. Letting yourself get hungry and going to a buffet is challenging. Letting yourself get hungry and going food shopping is…well, let's just say that you're not going to make the best food decisions! So, make a list, go to the store, and only buy what is on the list. It makes life so much easier.

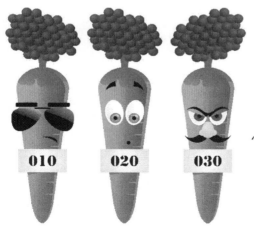

"Modern day foraging means finding the real food in a field of look-alikes."

CHAPTER 4

*"Needing to say 'no' to temptation
over and over again is very stressful.
A much better strategy is to
not be tempted at all."*

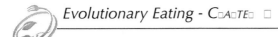

The Problem

"Thin Is In," But Our Habitat Is Fat

What is the perfect body for a woman? Is it related to a certain dress size? Or is it a specific number on the scale? Maybe it's a photoshopped picture of a movie star or model. One thing is for sure—for the vast majority of women, the perfect body is more slender than the one they are currently sporting.

Unfortunately, this is true even if you are one of those movie stars. The paparazzi are just waiting for the opportunity to snap their photo from a less-than-optimal angle, and sell it to the highest bidder.

Soon afterward, people flipping through those magazines at the grocery checkout are treated to the sight of ribs and hipbones as these same stars "get control." Why do we tolerate the endless parade of baby fat (or post-baby fat) turning into the fashionably thin and skeletal? The list is endless and occasionally even fatal. Do you think "baby fat" was on the death certificates of Karen Carpenter or Brittany Murphy, both dead at the age of 32?

But that's the world that we currently live in. Thinness is synonymous with beauty. Even slender isn't thin enough.

Coco Chanel is famous for her quip, "You can never be too rich or too thin." (Why are we taking advice from a woman with a name like a Yorkshire Terrier?!) The inverse is also true. Plump is ugly and more-than-plump is "disgusting." We don't hate our dog whose curves are a little generous, but we harshly judge ourselves, and everyone else—especially women.

You can see it everywhere—in magazines, on television, online, on every media venue you can think of. But that's not necessarily the problem. It is possible to be thin, but only if you have an environment that supports the behaviors that will make you thin. And the modern world is far, far from a thin environment.

Our world's cues conflict with our world views

Now, I'm not writing this to tell you that you should just accept the way you are. Truth be told, most of us want to be as attractive as possible. That's great. What I do want you to understand is that in today's environment, it is very difficult to be thin because although you may want to be thin, the world wants you to be fat.

Okay, that last part was intended to be tongue in cheek. The world doesn't actually want you to be fat. However, the world is making us fat through the environmental cues that surround us on a daily basis.

A cue is something that our senses perceive (for example, something we see or smell) that is relayed to the brain as a signal for action. The brain responds automatically (that means without your awareness) with a behavior or a set of behaviors.

So when you see candy on your desk, you might munch on it mindlessly. But when you see candy on your boss's desk, you "think twice" — and twice is often enough.

The problem is that the modern world is full of food signals that bypass the thinking process altogether. Here's a mouthful to chew over, one you might find hard to swallow.

Every day we make hundreds of food decisions, most of them "mindless." We aren't aware we're making them; we're simply responding to environmental cues. We used to have many cues that made us automatically NOT eat — we had food-free zones, designated meal times, and a mom who would raise hell if you raided the pantry, the fridge, or the food on the stove.

We now live in an environment that has an abundance of food cues. Cornell University food and behavioral researcher, Brian Wansink, conducted many studies on how elements in our environment make us eat more or eat less without our even being aware of it. Many of them are laid out in grim detail in his bestselling book, *Mindless Eating: Why We Eat More Than We Think.*

Wansink decided to take a careful look at the candy bowl. His research team placed a bowl of chocolate candies on the desk of every secretary in a particular office building. Half of the secretaries had a bowl that was clear, so the candies were always in view, and the other half had a bowl that was white, keeping the candies from being in direct sight.

Otherwise, there were no differences between the two kinds of bowls or their contents. Both sets of bowls were refilled nightly.

After two weeks, Wansink found that the secretaries that had the clear candy bowls ate 71% more chocolate candies than those who had the white bowls! Why did the secretaries with the clear bowls eat so much more?

Well, the candies were there for them to see throughout the day. These poor secretaries didn't just have a single cue — in the course of their day; the environment cued them over, and over, and over again. Every time they were cued, they were forced to make a conscious decision to NOT eat the candy because the human default position is to eat tasty food when we see it.

Willpower has its uses, but it must be applied judiciously. It simply won't work as a long-term strategy. How many times can one person say no? Once? Twice? How about 5, 10, or perhaps 20 times? After the 20th time resisting that candy, you may just give in on the 21ˢᵗ. Instead of feeling good about resisting, we feel terrible for giving in to the little voice that whispers, "Just one little piece won't hurt!"

Needing to say no over, and over again to temptation is very stressful. A much better strategy is to not be tempted at all.

That is what happened to the secretaries who had the white dishes. The candies were out of sight, and therefore they were out of mind. They had far fewer decisions to make because they couldn't constantly see the candies.

This is what I mean when I say that the world wants to make us fat. There are food cues all around us, and it eventually becomes too exhausting to constantly say "NO!" to those food cues. And it's not just visibility that we have to deal with. We also have to deal with other factors, such as convenience.

Wansink placed clear dishes of chocolate candies in the environment of a different group of secretaries. The candies were visible, but this time, Wansink moved the dishes around the room so that they were either more accessible or less accessible.

One week, a dish would be directly beside the secretary; the next week, it was in the desk drawer; and the following week, the dish would appear on the filing cabinet that was six feet away.

The results of this little experiment were pretty much what you would expect. When the candies were on the desks directly beside the secretaries, they ate an average of nine candies. However, when the dishes were on the filing cabinets six feet away, the secretaries only ate an average of four candies!

This is a perfect example of how small changes in the environment can create massive changes in behavior. That's why I emphasize over and over the importance of skill power over willpower—because the only thing harder than willpower is "won't" power!

Many more studies exist showing how our environment can alter what we eat. The environment in which we live has a dramatic effect on our eating habits, our food decisions, and how much we eat in general.

Perhaps the most harmful environmental change making us fat is the behavior I talked about in the "When" chapter— snacking. Historically, snacking was either not possible, or socially unacceptable, so we simply didn't think of not snacking as deprivation.

For example, 50 years ago, vending machines in schools were nonexistent. Only preschool children ate "snacks." Now we have legislation mandating that teachers allow students to eat in the classroom.

At the same time, we are screaming at schools to do something about the problem of our overweight and obese kids. How about a little change in environment?

We aren't fatter than previous generations because we are lazier. All humans are inclined to be lazy when offered the opportunity. We are fatter because we are relentlessly bombarded with cues to eat. If that wasn't enough (and it is), we have few eating skills. We are truly in over our heads.

Most of the problems began when we started producing surplus food in the 1970s. Since we were already eating the appropriate amount (overweight and obesity were rare), the food producers needed to find a way to get us to eat more.

They didn't really care whether we ate more or not—what really mattered to them is that we buy more, and keep buying more. It just happened to work out to their benefit, and our detriment, that the human default position is that when we overbuy food, we are also quite likely to overeat it.

What this means is that we need to become smarter about our environment. Anybody can be thin, but only if you understands how the environment is influencing you to become fat. Once you understand that, you can change your environment so it is making you thin instead of making you fat. This all begins with an extremely important concept called "habitats create habits." This concept offers a tremendous opportunity to create a real, lasting change in your life.

Our habitats shape our habits

The current food environment makes it very difficult for us to become skillful eaters. Cues are everywhere, and because they are everywhere, they are too hard to resist.

People talk a lot about willpower. But how can you say "no," 100, 200, or 300 times a day...every day...for the rest of your life!?

The reality is that you can't. It's the environment that dictates your habits and behaviors, not the other way around. Environment is much more powerful than willpower, because it's the habitats that create habits.

The way to allocate your willpower is not to resist eating, but rather to create boundaries where eating behavior can be framed in or fenced out. Then the habit will emerge naturally over time.

Direct your efforts towards your habitat, and healthy, thin decisions will become effortless. Habit change requires physical rewiring of your brain, which doesn't happen over-night, or from reading a book.

It takes many repetitions of the new behavior before your new-and-improved automatic decisions replace the old ones. Remember that the default human diet is the "seafood" diet—see food, eat food.

"Habitats create habits" means that your habitat, your environment, is what determines your habits. If you lived in an environment of skillful eating habits ,where everyone around you had eating competence, and there were reasonable social boundaries on our natural impulses, you would naturally develop more skillful eating habits.

But that isn't the situation in the modern world. So if the problem is that we are living in a "fat" habitat, a big part of the solution is designing your habitat in a way that helps you become an elite eater.

It seems so obvious, yet it's only the successful people that manage to do it. You can do that too. Let's begin by learning the next skill of *Evolutionary Eating.*

The Solution

Learn the "Where" Skill of Eating

The Fence and the Frame

Until very recently in human history, food was a specific ritual. There was a time to gather food, which was when you would learn where food came from. There was a time to prepare food, which was when you would learn about its complexities and varieties. Then there was time for eating, during which you would learn how to eat by eating with, and observing, those around you.

This was also a time to appreciate the food, and to develop your relationships with the people you were eating with. Where and with whom you were eating were so significant that the word we use today, "companion," comes from the Latin word "to break bread with someone."

That's where bonds were made, around the table. The "Where" was more than just a specific place to eat; it was the framework from which we would learn all of the other skills of eating.

Remember our little baby? The first skill of eating is to learn to stretch the interval between feedings. Newborn babies can only digest a single food, milk, and they must have that milk every few hours around the clock.

As the baby grows older, he or she can go longer without food, and can begin to handle a wider variety of foods. These foods are chosen by the baby's mother or some other adult.

Learning the skills of eating begins very early in childhood. Traditionally, the next important skill for a young child to learn was "Where" to eat. Babies are initially only interested in mom and milk, but by the time they are a year old, they are much more mobile and aware.

They have a strong drive to "be where the action is," and until very recently that action was commonly found at mealtime, where family and friends gathered to not only eat, but also talk and socialize.

Stop eating here, there, and everywhere

We gathered around the fire, and then we gathered around the table, to share the fruits of our labors and reconnect. We didn't eat anywhere and everywhere like animals; we ate at a designated spot—a "Where." Today, the abandonment of the "Where" has meant that we no longer have this all-important environment where we can learn the skill of eating.

Even worse, we have become lost because this important evolutionary and social touchstone of gathering for a meal has been polluted and diluted. The loss of our Where skill isn't just a blow to our health and weight—it's a blow to our humanity.

In a world where everybody eats everywhere…in the car, in bed, at the desk, on the phone, on the street…it can be very, very difficult to regulate your eating habits. Everywhere you look, there is always somebody eating. We have constant food cues; constant triggers that influence us to eat now, eat quickly, and just shove the food into our mouths so we can get back to our fast-and-furious lives.

Nobody slaves over a hot stove; there are no sacred mealtimes. Everybody is busy, busy, busy, so we fit in meals and snacks whenever, and wherever.

Distinguishing your designated eating place

Food marketers know we buy food that is convenient, so that's how they package it. If we didn't buy it, they wouldn't sell it.

So SLOW DOWN for a minute, and just consider how few foods today require a table. Chicken nuggets, wraps, rolls, yogurt in a tube are just a few of the things marketed to us today. There are hot dogs (invented so the vender wouldn't have to dispense gloves with his sausages), hamburgers and, of course, all those sweet drinks.

We can have candy of every description, nuts that don't have to be cracked or shelled, and chips with dip already applied. Even the traditional finger food, fruit, is now too inconvenient—who wants to deal with peels, or cores, or sticky drips when fruit roll-ups are so much easier and very tasty to boot?

So many things are pick-up-able with our fingers—fish sticks, cheese sticks, and potato sticks (French fries), too. If they make them, we buy and eat them.

We are in such a hurry that we can't even eat a bowl of cereal. Now we have cereal on the go, cereal bars, and cereal "smoothies." Our food isn't just processed and packaged conveniently; it's basically pre-chewed. All we have to do is swallow it. And swallow it is what we do over, and over, and over.

We mindlessly munch away, already thinking about the next bite, or the next meal, before we even deal with what is in our mouth.

The hard reality is the world out there is like the Indianapolis Speedway, and we don't even have a learner's permit. The only way around this is to create your own social norms by developing and sticking to some boundaries and limitations—otherwise known as fencing out and framing in.

Fencing out

Fence out "everywhere," and start eating "there." There is a single designated eating place. You might have to include a secondary designated eating place at work.

Anywhere that isn't the designated eating place is a food-free zone. Fence out your food-free zones. It's up to you whether you jump in with both feet, or take it a step out a time (fencing out the car, the bedroom, the break room, and other such places).

When we have a designated eating place, we eat a lot less, and we have a lot less food preoccupation because we are eliminating many eating opportunities. Our brains won't cue us to eat in a certain place if they have been trained to know we won't eat in that place.

The very first behavior we need to develop when learning the skill of where to eat is to distinguish our designated eating place. If you aren't eating there, you have ventured off into the fenced off "food-free zone."

Framing in

Fencing out helps we control food cues by making most areas food-free zones. Some people find that restrictive and unpleasant—especially in the beginning, when they experience an immediate sense of deprivation. Deprivation is a stressful feeling.

It is an important factor in the abysmal success rates of most "diets." One of the ways to counteract that feeling is to enhance the positive.

Since there are few things more wonderful in life than a special meal or treat, I train people to learn the Where skill of "framing in." A frame is designed to surround and draw attention to something special, like a beautiful piece of art. When you plan and prepare meals. When you enjoy them in the company of others. When you truly savor and appreciate every bite, you are "framing in."

An important part of the "Where" is to prepare. For a baby eager to join the rest of the family, the "Where" is obvious. For grownups wandering around a world that bears a striking similarity to Candyland, it's a bit more complicated (but not too much).

Pick a table, pull up a chair, plunk down a plate of food, and eat it. Believe it or not, managing utensils is a bit like riding a bicycle—you haven't forgotten how.

Freebies and food preoccupation

Whenever you eat in a place outside of your designated eating spot, your brain makes an association between the pleasure of eating and the place of eating. That place formerly a food-free zone now becomes a free-food zone.

Human brains love freebies — we love them even when we know they are not really free, and that we might have to pay for them later. Freebies are very reinforcing. In other words, when you eat everywhere, your brain will begin to cue you over and over, stronger and stronger, to eat and eat now.

This intense and persistent brain message is called food preoccupation. Food preoccupation is a relentless torture that will not go away unless you give in to it. But when we give into it, it comes back even stronger. Sounds a lot like addiction, doesn't it? That's because it is an addiction — food addiction.

Now, you might say that people don't need to smoke or drink or take drugs, but they do need to eat. That's true, but modern food is more inherently "addictive," and the modern environment is enabling (to use "addiction speak"). So take the first step that all recovering addicts must take, and remove yourself from the areas where you "abuse." It's a step in the right direction, and there is a reward — freedom from food preoccupation.

The importance of fencing off the food-free zones cannot be overstated. When you don't have a designated eating place, you always have to make a decision. There are only so many times that you can make the right decision when you are suffering from food preoccupation.

Learning and practicing the "Where" skills of fencing in and framing out means there will be an end to food preoccupation.

What use is being thin if you are plagued with constant thoughts of food? These basic rules and guidelines eliminate a lot of the "I want this/I shouldn't eat that" battles that you may have had with yourself. When you have a designated eating place, and you eat only at that place, eating anywhere else doesn't even come into consideration.

Once you have established your eating place, you can begin altering your general habitat so that there are fewer and fewer food cues to trigger unwanted eating behavior.

But a designated THERE place (preferably a table) is the first step. Because it sets the context for your entire eating behavior, it's critical for you to master this fundamental skill before you start trying out a whole lot of "variations."

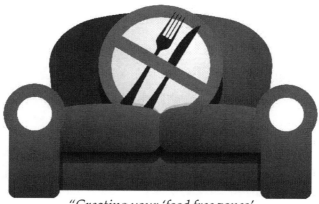

"Creating your 'food free zones'
will help you resist temptation."

The "WHERE" Skill of Eating

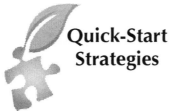

Quick-Start Strategies

1) Establish your designated food place

A designated eating place is going to "fence out" a lot of poor eating behaviors, and "frame in" a lot of good ones. It's really just too exhausting to constantly make the right decisions about food. But when you have a designated eating place, you really have only a few decisions to make. When you only eat in one place, your brain will learn you mean business and stop bothering you all the time.

2) Make sure that you have an "emergency meal"

An important part of the "Where" is "prepare." The hardest thing about designated eating places is that you sometimes have to plan in advance.

But life is hard, and food is easy. There will be times when you plans fall through. Be prepared by having a backup plan. You should always have one meal prepared in case of an emergency.

An emergency is usually when you are feeling extremely hungry, and you feel like you could eat anything! Maybe you've had a long day at work, and missed a meal. Maybe you're coming off a long flight, and have not eaten all day. Maybe you've just finished a long meeting.

Whatever the case, you need to have an emergency meal for the times that you just have to eat something, and simply can't wait to eat at your designated eating place. This will greatly reduce the chances of making a bad food decision.

The emergency meal should be designed so that you can bring it anywhere. Consuming this meal will temporarily reduce your hunger/cravings, and will put your mind in a better state until you get to a safer environment, such as your designated eating place.

3) Emergency meals shouldn't be treats!

I learned this one from my clients. (Thank you!) If you make your emergency meal something you really enjoy, you will find you frequently have "emergencies."

An emergency meal should be something you would only be interested in eating if you were very hungry. If you eat it too often, you will probably find that you start to like it more; make sure that you don't like it "too much." Also, make sure you don't have "too much" available. If your emergency meal is almonds and a fruit, make sure it isn't a jar of almonds and a box of fruit rollups. I recommend eggs as a good emergency meal at home. They are quick, nourishing, satisfying, and real food. In an "emergency," you aren't likely to get too fancy with them. Even if you are really hungry, it's hard to eat more than four eggs at a time. (But if you are still hungry and eat six, it's no big deal.)

4) Take control of your favorite foods (frame your eating)

When it comes to changing your eating behavior, you should never deprive yourself of foods that you love. Food is enjoyable and rewarding as long as you don't abuse it.

A "special occasion" designated eating place is a great strategy for frame in your certain foods. For example, let's say you love ice cream. It's a food that you can't keep in your house because you will just eat it all in one sitting, no matter how much of it is around!

Instead of never eating ice cream again, you can frame the experience of eating it—not by depriving yourself of it, but by only eating it when you go out for dinner. That way, the environment is safe—you only eat the portion served to you, and the ice cream is framed into a good behavior. Your lifelong success at weight control depends on how well you can handle the foods that tempt you the most, so it is critical that you do this step. And for goodness sake, when you eat your favorite foods, relish every bite!

5) Avoid eating in front of the television

It may take some time before you are only eating at your designated eating place, so a quick strategy to get you going in the right direction is to cut out TV eating.

Studies show over 40 percent more food is eaten while watching TV. According to Brian Wansink, "We often end up eating more because we simply eat to the pace of the program, or we eat until the program is over."

Anything that takes our focus off the food makes us more likely to overeat. If you have to eat in front of the TV, however, because it's one of the things that you really enjoy, then plan as much as you can. Dish out portions instead of taking the entire package with you.

6) Make television exceptions thoughtfully

For many of us, dinner is a lonely prospect. We must go home to an empty house or apartment. Our human brains are really distressed by this. For many people, the television is a soothing substitute for companionship. I definitely don't want you eating in front of the refrigerator or over the sink.

If you feel happier eating your meals in front of the TV set, make sure you employ some "framing in" strategies. Set your "table," and serve yourself your meal. Eat your meal, and put away the leftovers! But please, please do not snack in front of the TV, especially at night. This creates huge problems with leptin and insulin—a surefire way to get locked into fat-storage mode for a long time.

7) Keep your problem foods out of your home

You make life a lot easier for yourself if you keep your problem foods out of your home. This does not mean you should deprive yourself of these foods; however, if you can eliminate them from your sight, you can eliminate the constant visual cue of having them within your reach. Remember the secretary studies? Well, it's the same idea.

When the candy is always within view, you're going to want to eat it. So just put it away, and only eat it when you really want it, not just because it's there to eat.

8) Make overeating a hassle, not a habit

This is one instance where your laziness can come to your rescue. Numerous studies have shown that the more hassle it is to eat something, the less likely it is that you will eat it. For example, you would be less likely to eat ice cream if you had to walk to the store to get it than if you had some sitting in your freezer.

The convenience of a food, therefore, will usually determine whether you will eat it or not. Keep it in the kitchen, and not directly in front of you. This means that you will have to get up and walk to the kitchen to get more food. This little break will give you a chance to evaluate whether you are actually hungry, and it will reduce your risk of overeating.

9) Change your habitat

When it comes to food, it is a lot easier to change your environment than it is to actively change your behavior. We make, on average, 250 decisions every single day about food. Each time you have to ask yourself, "Will I or won't I?"

When you keep tempting foods around (and we all have our personal favorites), you are going to be food preoccupied. It's just too easy to get food.

Get it out sight, and if it is really tempting (or if you are vulnerable to nighttime nibbling or food binges), get it out of the house! It's even worse when you can see it. If there is a candy bowl on your desk, you will probably glance at it at least once every ten minutes. If you're like me, you will glance at it every ten seconds, and stare longingly at it every ten minutes. That's at least six times every hour.

Basic logic will tell you that some of those no's will eventually turn into yeses. Of course this usually happens in the form of, "Well OK, just this once..." Relieve yourself from this stress by changing your environment.

Get rid of all temptations that are near you. Remember the mantra, "Out of Sight, Out of Mind; In Sight, In Mind."

10) Make some rules about your home away from home

You might choose one designated eating place at home (usually the dinner table), and one at work (usually the lunch table). You then need to make some rules about eating outside of home and work.

- If I eat out, it must be at a table, such as at a restaurant.
- If I eat at a friend's house, it must be at his or her dinner/ kitchen table.
- If your life is really hectic (and whose isn't), at least think about the where and when. PLEASE Plan!

11) Remember "Not Yet" and "Not There"

Both the Where and When skills of eating deal with the problem behavior of snacking. Remember in the When chapter, I suggested you use positive language to deal with your brain. Human brains hate negativity and deprivation.

Instead of saying ,"I'm not going to eat," say, "I'm going to eat then" (designated time). Instead of saying, "I can't eat here," say ,"I'm going to eat there."

Now make sure you aren't lying. When you tell your brain you plan to feed it, don't go slithering out of your promise. That's a surefire recipe for revenge in the form of food preoccupation. Your brain will win in the end unless you play the game with cunning and skill!

CHAPTER 5

"We all learn to eat by watching others,
including TV people. There is no
getting around this! The only thing we
can control is who we allow
to influence our eating behavior."

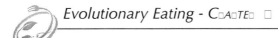

The Problem

It's Not About How YOU Eat, It's How Everybody Eats

Humans are lifelong learners. It is one of the unique aspects of our brains. One of the reasons we tend to forget that eating is a learned skill is that most of our learning occurs without our awareness.

Much of our learning occurs passively because we are hardwired to pay attention to what others are doing, mimicking and adopting the behaviors of the people around us. Most of the skills and behaviors we acquire throughout life are a result of our interaction with and observation of others.

One of the most evident of our characteristics as a species is that we are incredibly social. We not only pay attention to the behavior of others; we must, in fact, exert a continuous effort to ignore it. It's very hard not to "notice what someone else is noticing." We speak a certain language because that is the language that people spoke when we were young. We act a certain way because by interacting with the people in our environment that is how we learned to act.

181

How skillful we are at eating is also a reflection of the skill of the people with whom we ate and eat with today.

Human babies are born with almost no food instincts or behaviors—the two exceptions are we are born liking a sweet taste (the sweeter the better), and disliking a bitter taste (we spit it out). Even these instincts can be modified with learning— adults learn to like bitter foods like coffee, beer, and chocolate. We can also learn to curb sugar cravings, although they never really go away.

Mary Poppins was spot-on when she sang, *"A spoon full of sugar helps the [bitter] medicine go down."* One way to get children to like a new food is to "sweeten it up a bit," and then gradually decrease the sugar. An even more effective way of getting children to learn to like food is to give them dozens of opportunities to observe a trusted adult, a person they like, or a favorite character on television, enjoying a new food.

Everybody learns how to eat by looking at somebody else. There is no getting around this! The only thing we can control is who we allow to influence us and our eating behavior.

There is a good reason humans are wired this way. We are omnivores, and the natural world is filled with things that might be edible, but might also be poisonous. That's why the "What" skill is so important—all children must learn what foods are safe to eat.

But we learn the "What" skill from the "Who" skill. We do not learn how to eat by getting a degree in nutrition!

We are also strongly motivated by the actions of friendly and attractive people. We are particularly impressed (whether we want to admit it or not) by what "everybody" is doing.

Human beings are social—it is inherently stressful to feel separated from the group. As humans, we tend to eat like those that we eat with. To better understand this, let's take a look at Brian Wansink's analysis of yet another food study. In this study, researchers gave a participant some cookies.

Another person was instructed to be a "pacesetter," and eat a designated number of cookies. The results of this little experiment were always the same; whatever the pacesetter ate, the unsuspecting snacker ate also. If the pacesetter ate one, the snacker ate one; if the pacesetter consumed six...you guessed it...the snacker ate six.

Mirror, mirror (in your brain): Mirror neurons and behavior

Brain researchers have discovered one fascinating reason for why we are influenced to such an extent by other people.

Our brains are actually structured and designed to mimic the actions of others. This is done via neurons in our brains that are called "mirror neurons."

Mirror neurons are a very specific type of neuron. Neurons themselves have many functions, one of which is to communicate to your body how to move. If you want to move your hand, for example, these neurons in your brain "fire" a signal to the appropriate muscles in your hand; the muscles contract, and your hand moves.

Mirror neurons work by watching other people move. When you watch your friend eating a chocolate chip cookie, the mirror neurons in your brain "fire" as if you were eating the cookie yourself. By doing so, we can literally "feel" what the other person is doing, simply by observing them.

Mirror neurons and the media

Mirror neurons were only discovered and described recently. In 1992, a group of scientists in Italy were studying brain cells in monkeys, and were astonished to find cells that fired not only to signal a movement, but also when the monkey observed that movement.

It was a huge scientific breakthrough. We understood mimicry, which is "monkey see, monkey do." We had no idea that there was also "monkey see, monkey feel as if he is doing it himself" (even when he isn't!). Research in the area of mirror neurons is only beginning, but we know that humans have many more mirror neurons than monkeys do. More importantly, monkey mirror neurons do not fire when they are watching a videotape of another monkey.

In monkeys, mirror neurons only fire when the monkey watches a real monkey or human. However, this isn't true for humans. Human mirror neurons also fire when we see moving images of people on a screen.

The impact of modern media on our unconscious learning is significant. It is also brand new…just like the obesity epidemic. This new research demonstrates how vulnerable the human brain is to marketing messages. We used to learn how to eat from family, friends, and community—people who cared about our health and wellbeing. Guess who we learn from now?

The food industry isn't interested in the health of anything but its bottom line. We are learning to eat from an industry that exists to sell us food. So much for us being the "smartest" species. Maybe that's what is meant by "too smart for your own good."

Mirror neurons and emotion

Mirror neurons don't just affect our actions; they also have a profound impact on our emotions. Think about what happens when we watch sad movies.

They are called "tearjerkers" because we feel as if the tears are literally being jerked from our eyes. We are feeling the emotions the actors are portraying because our mirror neurons are firing as if we were experiencing those emotions firsthand.

Mirror neurons are one of the things that help us create a connection with somebody else. They are critical to our survival because they let us know the intentions of others simply by observing them. By activating the same neural pathway, mirror neurons make us want to do what the person we are observing is doing.

You are the average

One common observation in social psychology is that we are the average of the five people we spend the most time with. We behave, talk, walk, and even eat like them. A lot of this is due to mirror neurons. As you can imagine, this can either help you, or hinder you, when you are trying to change your behavior.

It will be nearly impossible for you to stop snacking if the people around you are constantly eating. Your mirror neurons will be telling you to snack because everybody else is doing it.

In the "Where" chapter, we learned that "habitats make habits." The people around you are a major part of your habitat. If you see somebody eating a chocolate brownie, the "chocolate brownie eating" parts of your brain get activated. Even looking at photos can activate these areas of our brains, and motivate us to eat. The more our mirror neurons are exposed to eating, the more powerful the brain activation, and the more intense the craving.

So, as you watch someone eating the chocolate brownie, your mirror neurons are telling your brain what's going on, but your pleasure centers are not happy because they are not getting any stimulation. This action ramps up your cravings even more, because now your brain begins to anticipate what eating the brownie would be like. You start to think how delicious it would taste. You think about how the texture would feel in your mouth and how you would feel if you just took a bite.

These are all the workings of your brain as it goes through your past experiences of eating foods similar to the chocolate brownie. You're doing well if you have still managed to hold out, but next come the biggest cravings. The greatest brain activation is achieved when anticipation is paired with a degree of uncertainty.

So you have one part of your brain telling you how delicious it will be (your mirror neurons are activating the movement patterns that are associated with eating the chocolate brownie) while your "rational self" is saying, "No, I have to stick to my diet!"

The food industry knows about mirror neurons all too well. That's why they place their food everywhere for us to see. They know that the more you are exposed to their advertisements, the more likely you are to consume what they are selling. They are also extremely clever in how they present their product. Have you ever noticed that food manufacturers advertise

555555555

their products by showing images of people consuming their products in a very fun and positive way? Manufacturers know that when you observe these scenarios, the areas of your brain related to happiness, and fun, and pleasure get associated with their particular food or drink.

Check it out the next time you watch an advertisement. And isn't it ironic that the actors are usually physically fit and very attractive? It's almost like consuming their product can help you with that too.

Fortunately, there is an antidote to the power of your mirror neurons. You can become a skillful eater. You can negate the effects of these negative influences in your life, and it doesn't require anything drastic like getting rid of your nearest and dearest. But you will have to make some changes.

In the previous chapter, I spoke about the importance of the Where skill, and how strongly our environment directs our food decisions. I introduced a new phrase, "habitats make habits."

The difference between habitat and environment is that your habitat isn't only your physical surroundings. A habitat includes your "people surroundings"—people who may be real or virtual. Habitats include the Who skill of eating, which is the next solution.

The Solution

Learn the "Who" Skill of Eating Surround Yourself With Skillful Eaters and Build a Community

A primary way that we learn to eat is by observing others. These people are called our role models. Either consciously, or unconsciously, we model their behavior.

We can have good role models, and not-so-good role models, and they all have different characteristics. For example, a bad role model for the "What" skill would be somebody who eats a lot of food forgeries, and not so much real food. A common role model for the current generation is someone who is "always on a diet."

Habitats make habits, and our habitat includes the people around us. When we establish good foundational habits, we decrease our vulnerability to poor role models, and media-marketing ploys. When we have those role models in place, we can develop other "Who" skills, but the first skill is to establish who has the eating skills that we want to have to use as our role model.

189

Common role models

Most of us are unaware that the way we eat is often formed in childhood, and largely based upon our role models. Most of the time we choose our role models unconsciously.

Primary role models are the ones to whom we have the most exposure. During the first few years of life, our role models are family members and caregivers.

As we grow older, this group grows to include friends, classmates, and co-workers. Some people influence us because we are repeatedly exposed to their behavior, but many times we choose role models, either consciously or unconsciously, from media personalities that we admire and want to emulate.

For example, men are greatly influenced by sports personalities because they admire them. That's why many of those same individuals promote food. They are paid to do so by the food industry because men will buy and eat what their favorite sports personality is eating.

If you need more convincing, look at the endurance of Wheaties cereal. It has been around for more than 80 years, and has always used the sports connection. You might not know that Ronald Reagan got his start in the 1930s as a result of his success as the "Wheaties announcer" for the Chicago Cubs. Talk about influence!

Women tend to be less interested in sports performance, and more interested in their appearance and their health, as well as the health of their families. Because female brains are wired to care more about people and relationships than performance, marketing messages that emphasize these things sell products.

There are many ways to enhance trust and authority, and they all work to enhance the value of the "Who."

We listen to what they tell us, but we don't realize that the visual messages carry priority in our brains. Our mirror neurons tell us that we should eat what this trusted person is eating, so we do. Not only do we eat according to what our role models eat, but we also act similarly to the way they do.

When did we begin learning the skills of dieting instead of the skills of eating?

Written history hasn't been around for nearly as long as human history, but we still have records from antiquity about the relationship between eating and weight. Of course, these words are "heavily weighted" towards the always pressing concern of not enough to eat. If you went to a doctor more than 100 years ago for your "weight," it was probably because you were losing weight.

Can you imagine what would happen if the doctor said, "Just eat more and work less"? Unfortunately that's analogous to what they say to people who don't know why they are gaining weight today: "Just eat less and exercise more."

Our society first began "counting calories" in 1918, when 45-year-old Lulu Hunt Peters published a breezy little book called, *Diet and Health: With Key to Calories.* Lulu was a Los Angeles physician who had struggled with her own weight for years.

Her little book, which sold about two million copies, mostly to women, bears a remarkable similarity to the Weight Watchers point system. At that time, no one had ever heard of calories, so Lulu included a helpful pronunciation guide in her book so the ladies could say the word accurately when they blabbed about it to everyone they knew. As far as ideas go, calorie counting was a real "lulu."

It took a while to catch on, but with the dawn of the new millennium, "dieting" became the standard way (or should I say "weigh") of eating for many Americans—especially women. On any given day, more than half the women in America are actively trying to "lose weight" on a diet.

A recent study in *Nutrition Journal* found that 83% of college-age women are on a diet, whether they are overweight or not. A large study in the *Journal of Pediatrics* found that 16% of boys, and almost twice as many girls aged 9 to 14, were already dieting. The study concluded that dieting in children leads to weight gain—not that you hear that on the news anywhere.

Children today are exposed to a mother who isn't just unskillful—she is often dysfunctional. Children are wired to learn about what foods are good (safe) and bad (unsafe).

It's hard to become skillful when so many people are exhibiting conflicting behavior—they say food is bad (meaning fattening), but they eat it anyway. They tell children they need to watch what they eat, instead of understanding that this isn't what people do.

Humans naturally watch what other people are eating! Unfortunately, many of these people are on television, exerting a profound and lifelong impression on the current generation.

The average American child watches between 25,000 and 40,000 commercials are year. More than half of these are related to food, and many of them are specifically targeted to children. Billions of dollars are spent marketing to children because it works; companies may spend billions, but they are getting a good return on their investment.

In the famous Doctor Seuss book, *Horton Hears a Who,* a Who has a very small voice. Modern day "Whos" don't just have a loud voice; they have a megaphone and message. And we are buying it without any conscious awareness.

You can't go back and relive your childhood influences, but you can change your habitat to learn new habits.

Adults can choose to surround themselves with more positive role models. They can even choose to become positive role models themselves.

It's hard to avoid the people in your life, and I am not asking you to shut them out—but I do suggest when it comes to the television that you "shut them off." Technology brought us television, but it also brought us the possibility of commercial-free viewing. The first step towards changing your "Who" habitat is to identify the potential problem areas, and avoid them.

It's not just the food they are selling us; it is also the image-and-diet plans. The fitness industry isn't as large as the food industry, but it is also very effective at capturing our hearts, minds, and hard-earned cash, while giving us very little in return in the way of long-term results.

When we listen to movie stars, or television-fitness-success stories, our brain gets a message loud and clear: "If they can do it, so can I! I just need the help of..."(whatever miracle solution they want to sell you).

It doesn't need to be direct either. The celebrity with the amazing body doesn't have to sell you anything—advertisers pay for the privilege of placing their ads in the vicinity of those gorgeous bodies. Our brains make all the connections for them. Marketers also know we are very susceptible to visual images. They take two photos of the celebrity, and post them side by side. One will be flattering, and the other will be not so much. If there isn't a dramatic enough difference, photo editors get to make the photos better or worse. The two shots are plastered side by side with a big splashy message saying, "Look how so and so went from flabby to fantastic in just six days!"

Celebrities are under tremendous pressure to look a certain way, and many of them have significant long-term problems with body image, body weight, and health. Many of them do not even enjoy food. This means that many of the people we base our eating habits on are not skillful eaters; they are skillful dieters.

Celebrities often have a habitat full of people who are paid to keep them thin and thinner, yet that sometimes isn't enough. We have all watched Oprah Winfrey, the richest and most powerful woman in media history, struggle with her weight. No one can say she lacks drive or self-discipline, but she has been unable to effect long-term weight management.

Oprah is a perfect example of a skillful dieter. She knows how to lose weight, but she doesn't seem to know how to stop gaining. She believes, like most people that "maintenance" is a slightly-less-restrictive diet. I believe her weight struggles are a testimonial to the ineffectiveness of dieting as a long-term strategy. The only way to stop accumulating weight, and maintain an attractive body, is through learning the skills of eating. One important step in that process is choosing the right role models.

Role models and support

To become a skillful eater, you need different people for different things. Often our family and friends are not the best role models, but they are crucial to our success because of the support and relief from stress they bring to our lives.

Sometimes even our closest friends and loved ones can unintentionally (or intentionally) act as eating-behavior saboteurs. Learning how to identify and deal with these people (while still maintaining the relationship) is very important to long-term success.

The second type of people we need is our eating role models. These are the people who we can model our skills of eating around. These are people who understand how to develop the skills of eating, and can answer our questions, or help us find our feet when we are going through difficult times. These are the people who know how to help us because they themselves have gone through the process of learning how to eat. You may be able to find these role models, for example, at farmers' markets and slow-food conventions.

Changing your behavior and your eating habits is just too difficult to do alone. You need help—not only from other skillful eaters, but also from those who are going through the same process as you. Eventually, you too will become a role model for skillful eating—a real role model, not a fake, photoshopped, celebrity spokesperson.

The "WHO" Skill of Eating

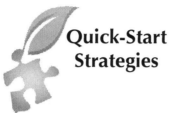 Quick-Start Strategies

1) Choose your role models

Who are you learning from—skillful dieters or skillful eaters? Most people believe that the best people to learn from are skillful dieters, but that just means that you are learning dieting techniques that will fail you in the long run.

A much better strategy is to model your behavior after people who have the skills that you actually need. It is the only place that I know where you can find people that are devoted to learning the skills of eating.

2) Have a pot luck

Just because you don't think you know any skillful eaters doesn't mean they aren't around.

It's nice to know that you have faraway Facebook friends, but sometimes a real face is what we are looking for. Make a real-meal date with a friend, or another family. Check out the organic food store, or even the organic food aisle. Look for local activities, like farm tours and apple picking.

An important part of the "What" skill is to learn where your food comes from. When you visit a local ranch that supplies grass-fed beef or pastured eggs, you expand your knowledge and your community. A great resource to find real food purveyors near you is *www.eatwild.com.*

3) Identify your saboteurs

The people we engage with on a daily basis have a tremendous influence on our behavior, particularly our eating behavior.

One strategy, therefore, is to only eat with skillful eaters. If this is too difficult (and it often is), try to identify any "saboteurs" in your life. These are the people who unintentionally influence you to eat either more food, or certain food, that you really don't want to eat.

Saboteurs can range from your well-meaning spouse, who would just like to go back to eating the old way, to your "frenemy," that colleague who feels competitive and stressed when others are able to successfully manage their eating behavior.

4) Make it public

The more people that you tell about the change you are trying to make, the more likely you are to change. The reasoning is simple. Once you tell people that you are going to change, you make it real. It is no longer just a thought in your head. Telling people about your change also makes you responsible and accountable.

Finally, telling people about your change makes it possible for you to seek their help and support. Once you do this, you can advise them about how best to help you throughout your change process. This factor alone will greatly increase your chances of success. Be sure to tell them what you intend to change is your behavior. Behavioral goals are far superior to short-term results goals.

5) Seek out helping relationships

Changing for good doesn't have to be difficult, but that doesn't mean it's quick and easy.

You will do a lot better if you have a support system in place. This can be anybody—a friend, a family member, a colleague, or somebody who has already achieved the change that you want. We all need support. It can be very difficult to change your eating behavior if you feel like you are doing it all on your own.

6) Help starts at home

Habitats make habits! I keep coming back to this concept because it really is that important.

When you are constantly exposed to poor eating skills, you have to constantly resist temptation. You can only use your willpower for so much, and so long. You may want to start with your family. Tell them about the skills you are learning.

A simple start would be to ask them to get rid of foods that are problematic for you, or at least make sure they are not storing them in plain view, and eating them in front of you. Eliminating this environmental cue alone can make a big difference.

7) Have a canned response
Because of the social nature of food, we are always going to be exposed to eating, and food pressure, throughout our lives.

It can be very, very difficult to say, "NO!" A much better strategy is to come up with a canned response to people when they are offering you food that you just don't want.

Some examples are:
- "Thank you very much, but I've just eaten and I'm very full."
- "Thank you very much, but I have some food sensitivities/allergies, and it's better if I eat food that I prepare at home."
- "Thank you, but I am fasting because I have a doctor's appointment tomorrow."
- "Thank you, but I had a dentist appointment today, and my mouth is still too sore to eat."

"Thank you, but no thanks—I don't like to eat when I'm not hungry."

 "Thanks, but I have dinner plans, and I don't want to spoil my appetite." (It's fine to "plan" for dinner at home!)

Of course, you could also just say that you are learning some eating skills! That may be more appropriate, and you could use your new knowledge to start a great conversation!

8) Understand status symbols

One of the reasons that restrictive diets are difficult to maintain isn't just that humans hate to be deprived. It's human nature to assign high status to those who get to eat the most and the "best."

If you are constantly experiencing feelings of unfairness because others get to eat and you don't, this markedly increases stress hormones. Stress hormones make it harder to get out of fat-storage mode.

9) And finally, get a coach

Having a coach can be critical for most people. A coach can identify your sticking points: what is holding you back, and what strategies are most important for your individual case?

You may like all of the strategies in this book, but what is the likelihood that you are going to use any of them? And if you do use them, are you going to continue to do so? That is what a coach can do for you. A coach can help you establish the best strategies for success, and can also keep you accountable to that success.

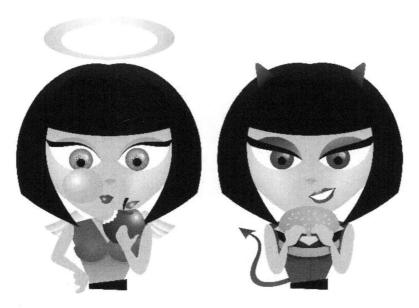

"Human beings are hard wired to notice and adopt the behavior of the people around them. When it comes to eating habits do you hang out with the wrong crowd?"

CHAPTER 6

*"Evolutionary Eating means
the application of skill power
rather than the exhausting and
ultimately futile use of willpower...
Why pick 'a physiology fight'
if you don't have to?"*

The Problem

We Know Our Body, But We Don't Know Our Brain

Decisions, decisions, and more decisions…the crucial point to keep in mind is that we actually make very few decisions—most are made for us. And who is this Machiavellian monster pulling our puppet strings? It's our very own brain.

The human brain has been referred to as a "kluge," an ill-assorted collection of parts assembled to fulfill a certain purpose. That purpose is to decide what we are going to do.

All human movement is purposeful, and our primary purpose is to survive long enough to pass on our DNA. We might go about this in an infinite variety of ways, and employ a huge number of actions. Even speaking (an action only humans can perform) is a purposeful movement, so deciding what to say is one way we plan what to do.

Animals differ from plants in a single fundamental way. Plants can make their own food from sunlight, soil, and water. As long as they are rooted in a favorable spot, they never need to "do" anything. Animals must eat food; that means we have to find, choose, and consume food, while avoiding "becoming food," in order to nourish our bodies and our cells.

Most of the food-related decisions that our kluge of a brain makes on a moment-to-moment basis are never relayed to our cortex, that newest part of the brain that makes us aware of our thoughts and decisions. Learning the skills of eating means that at least some of the time, your cortex will be in control.

Evolutionary Eating means the application of skill power, rather than the exhausting, and ultimately futile use of will-power. If you want to decrease your stress, you need to make sure all of your "brains" are in agreement. That is much less stressful. Why pick "a physiological fight" if you don't have to?

That's what a traditional calorie-restricting diet is—a physiological fight. Only a very small corner of our cortex cares what we look like naked. The vast majority of our brain is decidedly Darwinian. When it comes to the future of the species, survival, reproduction, and social connectedness are part of our genetic blueprint.

For millions of years, survival meant avoiding starva-tion, and fertility meant adequate body-fat stores in females. For humans, survival of the fittest was survival of the fattest. You must understand that automatic decisions are going to favor fat-storage mode—especially if there are any "starvation" or "summer" cues.

Summer is the season when days are long, and carbohydrates are abundant. Summer is the 7-11, where the lights are always on, and the shelves are bursting with sweets. Our DNA is screaming at us to stock up because winter is coming, Winter is coming!

Until electricity was invented, winter meant food was scarce, heat was what your body generated, and the best blanket was the layer of fat you wore until springtime.

Another way to describe the modern food environment is endless summer—one that cues our body to store up extra fat for a winter that never comes.

We go on a diet because we get fat and want to lose weight. Instead, we need to focus attention on the skills of eating so we don't get fat in the first place. Every human has a built in weight-regulating mechanism—when it is functioning normally, your appetite and your energy needs are in balance, and appropriate food decisions are made automatically. This is health—this is homeostasis.

When we eat all the time, eat food forgeries instead of real food, and overeat because normal satiety signals get blocked or distorted, we get locked into permanent fat-storage mode.

In fat-storage mode, you are drowning—you have to keep working hard to keep your head above water, but you can't do anything else. In fat-storage mode, your brain will relentlessly cue you to eat—you will be food preoccupied and hungry when you aren't eating, but your mind will mysteriously check out when you actually are eating.

When the brain goes on eating autopilot, it isn't hard to consume a container of ice cream, a giant bag of chips, or a whole plate of nachos. Like an alcoholic in a blackout, you don't even realize you did it until your spoon hits the bottom, your fingers come up empty, or you catch yourself prying up the last little bit of cheese from the edge of the plate.

In the previous sections, I discussed the When, What, Who, and Where aspects of eating. Traditionally, children learned these skills at the family table.

The "How" skill is one that we often pick up in a wider social context—it's much more related to custom, culture, community, and the classroom.

As Stephen Johnson, author of *Mind Wide Open: Your Brain, and the Neuroscience of Everyday Life*, states, "There is something powerfully human in the act of deliberately choosing a path; other animals have drives, emotions, problem-solving skills, but none rival our capacity for self-consciously weighing all the options, imagining potential outcomes, and arriving at a choice." Of course, most of the time, we don't really choose because most of our food decisions are not ones we make. They are ones that are made for us by the part of the brain that is on autopilot.

The key to changing automatic decisions isn't to try to alter the behavior after the fact—which is like putting the cart before the horse. It's much more effective to change the cues, so that our brain automatically makes a better decision. Automatic decisions are called habits. Changing our habitat is a great way to alter our habits; changing our How skills is another.

Most people make the mistake of manipulating numbers, like calories and grams. They also use numbers on a scale to weigh out portions, and watch their weight. This requires a tremendous conscious effort on the dieter's part. But almost no one can continue that forever, so the vast majority of dieting attempts may start off successfully, but ultimately end up as failures.

Instead of trying to eat less, and impose willpower on our eating behavior, we can change the unconscious cues in our environment so we automatically eat more appropriately for our needs. I call this happy, carefree state "homeostatic hum."

Think about it. We all want to be thin. We all want to look a certain way. So why can't we do it? Why do we do things we know we shouldn't do? Why do we do things we know we will regret? Hopefully, you are learning that our inability to stick to resolutions has nothing to do with willpower.

People who are stuck in fat-storage mode have tremendous motivation and desire to gain control of their eating, and their body shape. But they can't. And the reason is that they have the wrong goal (weight loss), and they are employing the wrong strategies (restrict calories intake and amplify calories burned) to get out of fat-storage mode.

They have failed to take in consideration that 800-pound gorilla in the room—the part of their brain that is automatic and unconscious, and has been shaped by millions, even billions, of years of life on the Planet Earth. Their misguided strategy is changing their mind, when they need to change the cues.

That, in turn, will automatically change their behavior, and eventually their habits. Since this is a lot less stressful, it also easier to continue to do this for the rest of your life. The rewards for this investment in diets and exercise are no longer necessary—instead, we get to eat and move in an enjoyable and rewarding way forever!

Although we all want to change our bodies, that's not what we need to focus on if we want to make real, lasting, sustainable change. You've learned throughout this book that you need to change your behaviors to have any chance of success.

Behavioral change means you are actually changing your habits. When it comes to your behavior, habits, thoughts, and emotions, your brain is the primary organ in charge. It doesn't make sense to have all this information about how our bodies work if we don't first understand how our brain works.

Since it's your brain that governs most of the other systems in your body (including how much you eat, and the amount of fat your body stores), you must learn how your brain works before you ever reach a sustainable weight.

You can't (and shouldn't) believe your eyes

The brain is the governing system of the body—it decides how much we need to eat, and how much fat we need to store.

The brain doesn't "know" these things. The brain bases its "policy decisions" on information that reaches it in the form of reports. The brain is always relying on second-hand information. The brain has no choice; it has no "eyes"…it can only use the information from the vision sensors, or eyeballs.

If that information is inaccurate or distorted, the brain must take action anyway. There is no "opt out" option. Automatic brain decisions that are based on faulty inputs result in "bad decisions." The long-term outcome is the brain will move from the poor strategy of ignorance, to the often worse one of ignoring. We call this situation—when the brain ignores input from the sense organs—"resistance." When you develop the skills of eating, resistance shouldn't be a problem. That's why it used to be rare for people to get fat—their sensors were accurate, and their brain responses were appropriate.

In our current environment, there are a lot of "tricks," many of which are profit-driven. In the When, Where, and Who chapters, we learned how the food industry and marketers use the media to signal us to eat anytime, anywhere.

Our brains quickly learn to respond by cueing us to eat all the time, and everywhere (food preoccupation). In the What chapter, we learned that food forgeries appear to our senses to be food, but are in fact just food-like substitutes that create tremendous problems in our bodies.

One of the craftiest strategies employed by the food industry is no more than a simple magician's trick. (That's actually good news because magic isn't really "magical" at all.) The food industry is a lot more Harry Houdini than Harry Potter. Learning the How skills of eating is both easy and effective.

Finally, some good news! If you know a little bit about how the brain works; you aren't susceptible to illusion, and can therefore beat the "How" tricks. Let's start with the visual system. When I ask people to define serving size, I get a lot different answers: a big spoonful, a cube of cheese the size of a pair of dice, 150 calories worth, two cookies, a piece of fruit...

The list goes on and on. The brain has an answer to the question as well: a default position that it will rely upon over, and over, and over, no matter how many diet books you read, food pyramids you follow, or labels you decipher (and decipher is exactly what you have to do).

The brain considers a serving size to be "the amount you are served." The brain doesn't know what to do when the cortex says a serving of meat is the size of a DECK of cards, and the grocery store says a modern chicken breast is rapidly approaching the size of a HOUSE of cards. It does, however, know that if you're not sure which way to go, bigger is usually better. At least, that is what the brain believes. Judging by the size of our butts, however, there appears to be a problem.

Our eyes and visual system have a built-in drawback. Like most miniaturized systems, they have to make a few trade-offs, one of them being that our eyes (and the visual part of our brain that interprets the input) don't know the true size of anything.

Vision is a perception, a guess. Our eyes make an educated guess about size by comparing objects, and by remembering past experiences. That means our eyes can't tell a two-ton truck from a toy truck replica unless there are other cues. Our brain can't tell how big a full plate of food or a hamburger is. A serving size is what we are served.

Until very recently, we were served food on 9-inch plates. Go to any flea market and see for yourself. If you buy a house with kitchen cabinets that were installed before the 1980s, chances are they won't even hold your dishes. Modern plates are usually at least 12 inches in diameter. Many of them are 13 ½ inches wide.

That's a big problem for us because the brain calls a full plate of food "a serving," and determines that you are full when you have finished that "serving." This begins happening to most humans when they are preschool-aged. They change from stopping eating when they are satisfied, to stopping eating when their plates are empty. For a long time, we thought this was because "ignorant parents" told their children about starving children in Africa or China, or cajoled them to join the "clean-plate club."

More recent studies indicate children will start to "clean their plate" based on many other cues. These are the "How" skills of eating. Putting it bluntly, when we throw out the plate and eat from a platter, it should be no surprise we have gotten fatter and fatter.

And the world finds itself having to shift around to make room for us. At the same time, the wall cabinets grew to accommodate our bigger plates, the seats in cars, movie theaters and even toilets have grown to accommodate our rapidly expanding rear ends.

In the last 50 years, plate size has increased from an average of 9 inches to 12 inches or even 13 inches, at the same time our waistlines have grown by 6 inches.

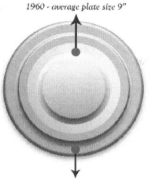

1960 - average plate size 9"

2010 - average plate size 12"

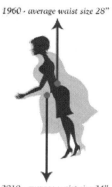

1960 - average waist size 28"

2010 - average waist size 34"

It all comes back to how our brain works to create our perception of the world. The human brain makes very predictable errors when it comes to perception. Scientists call them "optical illusions." Magicians call them "magic." Marketers call it "money in the bank."

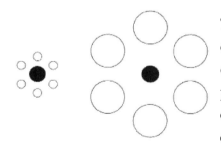

Take a look at the two black circles in this picture. Which circle is bigger? Normal people think that the circle on the left is bigger than the circle on the right.

In reality, the dots are the same size, but our brains perceive them to be different because we make sense of the world by comparison. The circle on the left looks much bigger because it is large compared to the smaller circles around it. The circle on the right looks much smaller because it is small compared

215

to the circles around it. So what? Well, sometimes three small inches makes a huge difference: A 12-inch plate holds almost twice the food of a 9-inch plate.

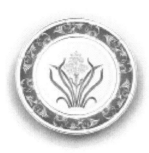
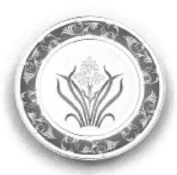

That little change in diameter makes a big change in how much food you will actually eat. A 12-inch plate (which isn't even a big plate today) has 77% more surface area than a 9-inch plate, and holds about twice as much food.

Unfortunately, the typical human brain doesn't just struggle with percentages and proportions during middle school math class. It prefers to ignore symbols and numbers because they are difficult. Human brains are fond of simple things like 100% full or 100% empty. This lazy tendency doesn't serve us well, either for math tests or serving sizes.

When it comes to eating from a 9-inch plate or a 12-inch plate, the typical brain doesn't feel any more or less full when it eats a plateful—even though the big plate contains twice the amount of food.

Portion distortion

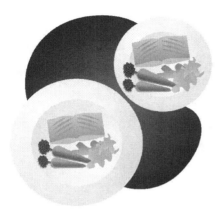

Dietician Dr. Sandra Frank asked the following question: *Which plate has more food?*

Most people looking at these two plates will think there is more food on the plate on the right. We perceive it that way because of how we use comparison to create our perceptions. The reality is that there is exactly the same amount of food on each plate.

There are two primary ways this distorts how much we will eat. The first is portion distortion. The food on the 12-inch plate looks like a small amount of food compared to the smaller plate, so we perceive it as being less than one portion.

Again, the whole notion of portion is just a perception in the first place. We can eat the entire portion of food that is on the plate and still feel hungry because the amount that we ate was less than one single portion.

Then we go back for seconds! Contrast that with the "used to be the norm" 9-inch plate. There is very little "empty space," so we perceive it as one full portion. We can eat the exact same amount of food, but this time feel satisfied, simply because our brains' perception has changed!

There have been many studies on how external cues influence our eating behavior. Most of these studies suggest we have a very hard time telling how much we are eating, or how much we ate.

People aren't necessarily lying when they misrepresent their food intake. Much of the time they aren't consciously aware of it. The brain tells us when to eat and when to stop eating, a complex and multifactorial decision.

We have all heard of someone with Alzheimer's disease or a head injury who asks, "When is lunch?" moments after they finished eating it. The only difference between us and that person is the level of brain confusion.

The stomach doesn't tell you to stop eating; the stomach doesn't signal fullness. The stomach and the other body sensors tell the brain, and only then does the brain decide to relay the message to "us," our conscious awareness. Until we are consciously aware of something, we cannot possibly make a "conscious decision" to stop eating.

We can learn to spot the tricks

Look at these two lines.

Which line is longer?

Virtually everybody thinks that the vertical line is longer by about 18% to 20%. However, both lines are actually the same length.

See...well, you can't really "see"; that's the point. We perceive based on many cues, not just on reality. Because the brain is blind, it doesn't see; it perceives. It makes a "best guess" based on incoming information.

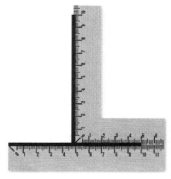

The difference between the image above and this image is that the one below has more information in the form of a ruler, something we LEARN is a reliable way of measuring. We can LEARN to avoid overeating cues by training in the How skills of eating.

Hopefully, you have learned that it doesn't really matter how much you know about calories, or portion sizes, or any other dieting metric. Our brains are what really count, so we need to shift our attention to how our brain works. Once you learn to make small changes in How you eat, you send an "I'm full" report to your brain much sooner. When your brain is so informed, it will respond with an "I'm finished" report.

This will go a long way towards reducing how much you eat without feelings of deprivation. Your brain isn't really happy about "eat less." So trick your own brain—it's easy once you learn and apply the How skills of eating.

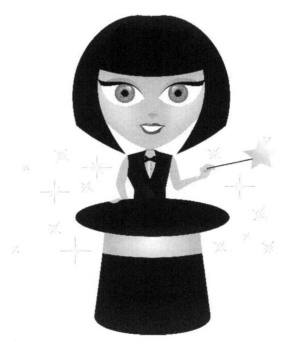

"Eating is like magic…It's all about illusion!"

The Solution

Learn the "How" Skill of Eating

One of the most profound scientific discoveries of the new millennium is the revelation that the brain, which was thought to be fixed and static after childhood, is actually capable of physical (anatomical), and physiologic (functional) change throughout the entire adult period.

Neuroscientists call this phenomenon neuroplasticity, probably because they love to impress people with big words. I call it "BrainChanging" because it means the same thing. (Neuro means brain; plasticity means changeability.)

In the "How" skill, we learn how our brain works in relation to how we eat, and how much we eat. We use the principles of neuroplasticity, or BrainChanging, to help people learn new-and-improved skills and habits.

Out of all of the eating skills, the How is perhaps the most deceptive because it is the one that we tend to pay least attention to. Even those who care little about their food, spend some time making choices about What they eat, When, Where, and Who they eat with. But very few people know the impact that How they eat has on their eating behaviors and decisions. The good news is that it is actually quite painless to make many of the How changes and become a more skillful eater.

How to eat less without suffering more

There is no question that if you want to become thinner, you are going to need to eat less.

What most people don't realize, however, is that the way you eat less is not by imposing draconian measures on yourself, and then implementing those measures with willpower. That strategy is ineffective and unpleasant.

A much better option is to learn about the brain, and then use that knowledge to your personal advantage. When we know how our brain works, we can structure our environment in such a way that we automatically eat less because we feel satisfied sooner. That allows our brains to send those desirable stop-eating signals. Hooray!

I am very grateful for the numerous, well-done studies, conducted by Dr. Brian Wansink at the Cornell Food and Brand Lab. He's been called the "Sherlock Holmes of Food," and the "Wizard of Why" (we eat, and eat, and eat) for good reason. Frankly, without Dr. Wansink's hard work and dedication, this How chapter wouldn't be nearly as helpful.

I have spent a lot of time discussing perception and the brain. Perception is an end result, or interpretation, based on information delivered to the brain by our senses, combined with past experiences (learning).

Perceptions are a "best guess" only. We never base decisions on all of the information because we don't pay attention to all of the information. If we didn't have these attention filters in place, we would quickly become overwhelmed with "too much." This is what happens to children with autism; they have to "tune out" because they don't have an ability "turn off" much of their sensory input—everything is important.

Our brains are always making guesses based on the "evidence." Our brains consider some "evidence" to be much more convincing.

As many of us have learned on television shows, like *Law and Order,* human brains love visual evidence, like "eye witnesses," no matter how often they are proven to be unreliable. Fortunately, we now have the much more dependable and accurate DNA evidence.

This is the problem with "intuitive eating" diets. Many fitness gurus have embraced the idea of eating in response to internal body cues as an alternative to traditional diets. I believe that idea actually trades a bad strategy for an even worse one.

First of all, we don't just have internal cues to contend with—only babies do. We live in a world and environment to which we are designed to respond to external cues, and pretending we don't respond to them is ludicrous and irresponsible.

Furthermore, most of us have immature, or even infantile, eating skills. You don't give children the keys to the car, and you shouldn't give unskilled eaters a big plate at a buffet.

Why should you listen to your body when your body (actually your brain) is obviously not fully prepared to handle that responsibility? Eventually, it will be appropriate to eat "intuitively," but first it is necessary to develop a minimal level of eating competence. Since we know we can't believe our eyes (intuition), we have to make an effort to process some of the evidence.

You have been judged and found guilty of being "just a normal human"

We tend to rely much more on our eyes as an indicator of our satiety than our stomachs. When we can see the food we are eating, we tend to eat less than if we don't. But human stomachs are quite interesting. Relying on them is risky because the human stomach has an amazing ability to "stretch the truth."

At rest, our stomach holds about 75 ml or 5 Tbsp. But by relaxing the fibers hormonally, the stomach easily expands and can hold up to four liters of food—that's more than 50 times more than an empty stomach! We evolved this capacity for the same reason anacondas did — so that when food was available, we could gorge. Our ability to stuff ourselves with food, and store it as fat, was very important to our survival as a species. Just because food is abundant for the first time in history doesn't mean our genetic makeup can change overnight.

So when food is available, we eat it. When you serve yourself large portions or, even worse, "bottomless" portions, your default setting is to eat until you physically can't eat anymore. Who hasn't experienced the physical discomfort of overeating? Our neurological system doesn't just fail to tell us we are full; sometimes, it doesn't even tell us when we are overfull. We have to educate our backup systems. That's the How of eating.

Where did those wings fly off to?

In a recent study, Cornell researchers invited a group of grad students to an all-you-can-eat Buffalo Wing feast at a sports bar on Super Bowl Sunday.

The students were instructed to eat as many wings as they wanted throughout the game. The only other instruction was that they had to leave the chicken bones on the table at which they were seated.

During the game, the researchers had the servers clean up half the tables, but on the other half, they left the grisly remains to pile up as the game progressed. Nearby Buffalo is the home of the chicken wing, so the researchers weren't surprised that the students attacked them with enthusiasm. However, they were quite surprised to find that cleaning away the "evidence" had such a dramatic impact on consumption.

The students who didn't have to "face the evidence," ate 40% more wings than the students who had to look at the growing pile of cast-off bones.

When it comes time to remember how much we ate, our brains are very inaccurate. Over and over, studies show that people underreport what they have consumed — to researchers and to themselves. They aren't lying. It's just the way our brains work.

In other studies, researchers found that when people pre-plate their food, they eat 14% less than when they take smaller amounts and go back for seconds.

The reason is the same. When you put everything on one plate, you can see exactly how much you are eating, but when you nibble throughout the day, there is absolutely no evidence of what you ate, so you just forget that it ever happened.

Can you see why the whole notion of calorie counting is so problematic? Your brain doesn't count calories. It has many other more reliable means of making sure you get enough to eat.

It takes skill power, not willpower, to gain the advantage instead of those extra pounds.

We like the lion's share (the bigger one)

The brain estimates whether a meal is likely to be satiating (filling us up enough to last until the next meal) based on volume.

This principle was studied extensively by Dr. Barbara Rolls, and reported in her bestselling book, *The Volumetrics Eating Plan: Techniques and Recipes for Feeling Full on Fewer Calories.*

The principle of volumetrics is quite simple. If you add high-volume foods to your meal, you will make it look like you are eating a lot more, although the amount in terms of the energy you are eating will not be that different at all.

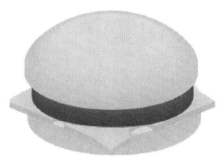

There are a few ways that you can do this. The first way is by making your portion size look a lot bigger. Take this burger for example: if you eat this and feel satisfied, great, you have established what a portion size is for you.

If, on the other hand, you are still hungry after eating this burger, you could add volume using light foods, such as lettuce, tomato, onions, or cucumbers, to make the burger look something like this:

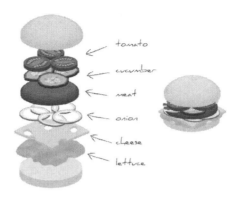

Because you are eating a burger that looks a lot bigger, you will be more satisfied than if you ate the first burger above. This is just another way that our eyes trump our stomachs when it comes to the perception of what we are eating.

Another way you can use volumetrics is by replacing heavier foods with lighter foods. Again using a burger example, you could replace an 8 oz burger patty with a 4 oz burger patty, and then fill up the rest of the roll so that it looks like there is an 8 oz patty in there. Add lots of the high-volume, light foods like lettuce, onion, and tomatoes to do this. You will be just as satisfied, while actually eating a lot less.

We pay much more attention to external cues like the size of food than we do to internal cues, such as how hungry we feel. How we present our food makes a big difference in whether we are likely to feel satisfied.

When we change the way our food is displayed, even when we do it ourselves, we change our perception about whether or not it is enough. For example, two hardboiled egg halves might not be enough, but fan out the slices of egg and we might very well feel it is plenty because this looks,

like this: instead of this:

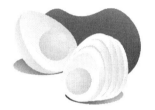   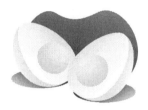

When it comes to eating scripts, you have to learn to "improvise"

Eating scripts are the personal habits or rules we learn in childhood that usually stick with us for life. Most of our eating scripts tend to make us fatter—especially if we are American.

Traditionally, lean cultures, like Japan, France, and Italy, have skinny scripts. For example, in Japan, the eating script *Haru Hachi Bin* means to eat until you are 80% full.

The American script tends to be eating until you are finished or, even worse, eating until you can't eat anymore! Maybe that's why the average American woman is 163 pounds, and the average Japanese woman is about 114. Perhaps if we ate from the 80%-full script, we wouldn't weigh 40% more.

The "HOW" Skill of Eating

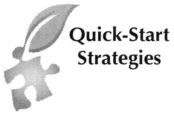

Quick-Start Strategies

1) Learn how your brain works

Evolutionary Eating uses brain changing principles to train the fundamental skills of eating. BrainChanging for adults differs from the process for children. BrainChanging involves competition for high-priority areas.

A simple (maybe too simple) way to look at it is that a child's brain is a mostly empty hard drive and an adult's brain is a mostly full one.

We need to get rid of a little "cognitive clutter," and replace old habits with new ones. This doesn't happen when you change your mind or read a book. This happens when you use the BrainChanging recipe of mindfulness, movement, and mood. We must focus our attention on the behavior we want to change, and make sure that it's personally relevant and meaningful.

The brain values purposeful and personal goals, so we must be mindful of what we want to change. The brain also values movement; you must physically practice new behaviors in order to make a new habit.

Finally, the brain isn't really open to change when we feel stressed, scared, or unhappy. A positive mood releases reward chemicals in the brain. We often undertake traditional diets with a negative mindset, feelings of deprivation, or unfairness, and often body hatred.

When you are practicing your new skills, remind yourself that you are training for life—and smile.

2) Learn a lesson from Goldilocks

Eat from a plate that is "just right." That means either 8.5 or 9 inches in diameter, including a border. Don't make the error of using a 6- or 7-inch dessert or salad plate. The brain figures out right away that it isn't meal-sized, and you will likely walk away too hungry, or go for seconds. Use the right-size plate.

3) Use a ruler!

Preferably, use a ruler you can carry with you. My handspan is 8 ½ inches, and I usually carry my hand around with me. One of my clients carries a folded paper plate in her purse, as most of them are 9 inches. The small ruler also comes in handy when you go grocery shopping.

We are so accustomed to oversized portions that most people don't realize that a modern-day chicken breast barely fits on a 9-inch plate. Learn to shop for food that fits, then prepare and plate it so it looks pretty! Take time to admire it before you dig in.

4) Save seconds for special occasions!

Generally, I'm not a fan of diet books, but I do like *The No S Diet*, by Reinhard Engels. The No S diet is very simple — No Sweets, Snacks, or Seconds on any days except those that start with the letter S: Saturdays, Sundays, and Special Days (your birthday).

I'd rather people drop the snacking altogether, but Reinhard wrote an excellent book, and made some great podcasts on his blog at *www.everydaysystems.com*.

Decide in advance that you are only going to eat one plate of food. When you start out, you might want to pile it up to make sure you "get enough." Once your brain starts to trust you, you will probably find this visually looks like too much food, and start plating appropriately.

5) Buy small packages

People tend to eat 20% to 25% more when they eat from large packages. For snack foods, it's even worse. When two groups of volunteers were given two different-sized bags of M&Ms,

the first group (half pound bag) ate an average of 71 M&Ms. The second group was given a one pound bag of M&M's, and they ate 137, which is almost twice as much. So if you are going to have treats, make sure you buy them in small packages!

6) Utensils, bowls, and cups count too

People eat with their eyes, not with their stomachs. If you give someone a meal on a big plate, her brain automatically registers that as one portion.

You know from previous experience that you are usually full after eating one portion. So you will eat the whole plate of food, just because you think that it is one portion.

The same can be said for bowls, glasses, cups, forks, knives, and whatever you eat food with. These have grown in proportion to the plate size. Shop around for more "fitting" tableware.

Here's another example of American supersize mentality. The Swedish company IKEA was mystified by the American practice of buying vases in sets of 4 or 6. They were surprised to find out that we thought these large containers were glasses! Remember the vertical-line illusion. Even very experienced bartenders are susceptible to this one. They consistently over-poured when using a short, fat glass—37% more on average. And these are professionals. Use tall, skinny glasses for your drinks. Champagne, anyone?

7) Boozy brains make bad decisions

The first thing that happens when you drink alcohol is that you lose your judgment. When under the influence, people tend to overdrink, overspend, and overeat. They don't remember it either.

When you have a before-dinner cocktail or glass of wine, be aware that you will naturally, and automatically, eat more. Be careful, or cut out the booze altogether.

8) Don't blow it on the weekend

When you are learning a new set of skills, you must remember that the old bad habits aren't gone yet. BrainChanging is like making a new road in your brain; to use a new pathway, you must obliterate the old one.

A mistake people often make is reverting to old habits on the weekend. They sleep in, miss breakfast, nibble all day, and drink too much. Try to stick to your game plan guidelines during the weekend. You'll find it is much easier, and more effective, in the long run.

9) Replace bad behaviors with good ones

To maintain a healthy weight, you will want to replace bad behaviors with good behaviors. For example, if you are bored, instead of eating, go for a walk, and listen to your iPod. If you must nibble when you cook, nibble on vegetables instead of cookies. If you always head to the fridge when you come home from work, interrupt that by doing something different, like taking a shower, or calling a friend.

The important point here is that you change negative behaviors by replacing them with positive ones. Again, the key is to become aware of your negative behaviors because you can't change something you don't know exists.

10) Add light foods with high volume

This is a great tip from the *Volumetrics Eating Plan.* Portion distortion can also be manipulated within the food itself. For example, let's say that you typically drink a 12-ounce smoothie, and it satisfies you. Now, if you drink an 8-ounce smoothie, you probably won't be as satisfied. However, if you make the 8-ounce smoothie LOOK like the 12-oz smoothie, by adding air to it, and letting it sit longer, it will make you just as satisfied as if you drank the 12 ounces–even though the smoothie is just 8 ounces! Remember this important point. People eat with their eyes, not with their stomachs.

So if you can add high-volume foods to your diet, you will feel just as full, even though you will have actually eaten quite a bit less.

11) Chew your food

Chewing your food does a number of important things. First,

by chewing your food more, you will eat more slowly. This will give your brain a chance to register the amount of food you have eaten before you eat more than you actually want.

Secondly, by focusing on chewing your food, you will be encouraged to buy food that actually requires chewing. This means you will be eating real food, and fewer food forgeries. Food forgeries are palatable—they are easy to chew and swallow. This is good for the bottom line of the food manufacturers, but is likely to make the line at your bottom a lot bigger!

12) Wear a belt

It might surprise you that the main reason people gain weight in prison isn't fattening food or lack of exercise—it's the baggy orange jumpsuits that hide the average pound-a-week gain. It's like you were pregnant, and didn't even notice!

The food industry isn't the only one contributing to our "fatness"; the fashion industry is in cahoots. They have banished the belt, and started making clothing loose and stretchable. They call the new fabric spandex, but they should probably rename it EXspandex! Since losing abdominal fat is an attractive AND healthy body-shape goal, try ditching the scale and bring back the belt.

13) Pace yourself

Many cultures place food and meals at the center of their cultural and social activities. Why aren't they fat? They often serve food in small courses. They pay attention to each dish. Food isn't just about fueling up as fast as you can so you can get on to better things. Food is the better thing. That's why restaurant critics aren't fat either. Slow down and make meals a special occasion. You do deserve a break today—but that doesn't have to mean fast food. One great strategy is to use a "speed bump."

Mentally divide your plate of food in half or even thirds. When you have finished the first half, pause and ask yourself, "How do I feel? Am I still hungry? Am I full?"

The food script in France, where people love their food, is to eat until you are no longer hungry, not eat until you are full. You can redefine the word "satisfied," and you don't even have to learn to speak French. But if you're interested, the French word for satisfaction of the senses is *plaisir*, which also means pleasure. Cultivate *plaisir*.

14) Some salads aren't so skinny

Many of my clients think salads are a great choice. It certainly is a good idea to get plenty of real-food veggies. The problem is that they put salad dressing, cheese, croutons, and meat in the salad to make it more filling. Salads in restaurants often have more calories than a complete steak dinner—including a dessert!

Eat vegetable salads made of leaves, and dress them with olive oil and vinegar or lemon juice. Use plenty of salt and pepper. Gradually decrease the amount of dressing over time. Make a little dressing go a long way by tossing the leaves in a big bowl before you dish out a serving.

15) Eating out can be challenging

Eating out is much more common these days, and it is probably an important factor in the current obesity crisis. You don't have control of your food when someone else prepares and serves it to you.

The Spice Girls might have asked, *"Just tell me what you want, what you really, really want,"* but the food vendors already know.

We like huge portions of tasty, highly palatable food— that means lots of chemicals, unhealthy fats, and gargantuan portions.

I consider eating out to be very challenging for unskilled eaters, but for many of us there really isn't another good option. There are many dining-out strategies, but here are a few down-and-dirty tips:

🖋 ALWAYS eat off a plate.

🖋 Try to use utensils to eat everything.

🖋 Get the doggy bag first! Divide your meal in half, and put the rest in the bag before you begin eating.

🖋 Avoid beverages with calories.

🖋 Order off the kids' menu. A Happy Meal is actually the appropriate size for an adult—put it on your 9-inch plate and see!

And most importantly…

🖋 DON'T EAT THE BREAD. They give it to you for "free" because when you eat the bread, you are more likely to eat more, drink more, and order the dessert. Please give the bread a pass! (That goes for the tortilla chips, too.)

CHAPTER 7

*"All humans are emotional eaters.
We all eat food, and everybody
gets a release of reward chemicals
in his or her brain for doing so."*

The Problem

We Eat for Stimulation Instead of Eating for Nourishment

Why do we eat more than we want to? Why do we eat things that don't even taste good? Why is food so addictive? Why can't we just eat what we know we should eat?!?

The answer is that food is emotional. Emotional Eating is something that everybody has heard of, yet it has no formal definition.

Many people describe it as the process of eating certain foods that make them feel better. Some people eat when they are sad or anxious. Others eat when they feel stressed out, while, for many, the cue to eat may come when they are bored, lonely, angry, or depressed. Although the reasons may vary, the results are the same...

People eat food because it makes them feel better

Food makes us feel better because eating, in general, creates good feelings in the brain. Foods that make you feel extra good are said to be highly hedonic, and are typically sweet,

243

salty, and high in fat. Since these hedonic foods are rare in the natural food, it has traditionally been difficult for us to overindulge in them.

In the natural world, sugar comes packaged in a stick! It takes a lot of labor to extract it from sugar cane. Sugar is also present in fruits, but the fruit season used to be fleeting—you don't get fat by overindulging in strawberries and blueberries a few weeks out of the year.

Everybody is an emotional eater

What people don't understand is that EVERYBODY is an emotional eater. We all eat food, and everybody gets a release of reward chemicals in his or her brain for doing so. For example, almost everybody has stuffed him- or herself so much that it nearly made him/her sick.

Some people do this habitually; their internal script is to eat until they feel distended. But even people without this problem will occasionally overeat or binge to the point of discomfort.

Why do we let ourselves do this? We do it because we are human, and all humans are emotional eaters.

Even in the absence of hunger, our brains will keep rewarding us with feel-good chemicals as long as we are chewing and swallowing. That's why it's sometimes hard to stop—our brain wants us to keep eating.

244

Don't forget that for most of our existence, there was no way to store food. When food was available, we needed to eat it and wear it. Food in your saddlebags spoils. Food ON your saddlebags lasts all winter long.

The real problem develops when our brains start to associate certain emotions, places, or behaviors with eating. When that happens, we develop repetitive behaviors, and always eat under certain circumstances.

In essence, people create a script that is imprinted in their brains, and this behavior becomes so routine that they respond even before they are conscious of a stimulus. For example, "Every time I get stressed, I eat ice cream." That is why sometimes you find yourself scraping the bottom of the ice-cream container without even realizing you have eaten anything at all!

This process is called "conditioned learning." Basically, conditioned learning means that you have trained your brain to react a specific way under specific circumstances. Emotional eating when you are stressed, or angry, or lonely, or sad is a learned behavior that you have created in your brain through association. It is a conditioned response.

Emotional overeating is a habitual behavior

If people want to change, they can't rely on willpower and short-term strategies, like diets and weight-loss programs.

Real change requires that we change the underlying factors that are making us overweight—our behavior and our habits.

The habit of eating when you are bored, or sad, or anxious is not "emotional eating." Remember, we are all emotional eaters, but we are not all overeaters. Overeating is a learned behavior.

Every time you eat when you are angry, you strengthen the "When I am angry, I eat" habitual response. Conversely, every time you do not eat when you are angry, you weaken that response. This process is called neuroplasticity, or BrainChanging, and it is how our brains change in response to the actions that we take.

Emotional eating has received a bad name. The truth is that eating is supposed to be emotional. Humans are supposed to enjoy our food and feel better when we eat. Skillful eaters love food because food is meant to be joyous, pleasurable, and life-sustaining. Enjoying our food isn't the problem. We get into trouble when we eat because we want to make a bad feeling go away.

Eating for stimulation

Our brains are structured to give us a lot of reward chemicals when we eat food. These chemicals are called endogenous neurotransmitters, which can be translated to mean "self-made drugs." Drugs, you say!? Yes, your brain makes drugs, and lots of them!

We are all born with an internal pharmacy, as well as our own private pharmacist. When you write yourself illegal prescriptions in the outside world, you might land in jail. When you write yourself prescriptions in your internal world, you might land in hell—the hell of food preoccupation and perpetual fat-storage mode.

Typically, when we think of drugs, we mean illicit or illegal substances that we ingest or inject. In medical terms, these would be referred to as exogenous drugs. But we now know that we also have endogenous drugs.

For the sake of simplicity, let's call the exogenous drugs, "man-made" drugs. So we have "self-made" drugs, and "man-made" drugs. An example of a "man-made" drug is cocaine. This drug induces your brain to release a neurotransmitter, a feel-good chemical called dopamine. Dopamine is released in the brain when we experience something as pleasurable. Smoking, snorting, or injecting cocaine produces a similar feeling of euphoria.

So while dopamine is a "self-made" drug that makes us feel very happy, cocaine is a "man-made" drug that does the same thing, but by "cheating." Both cocaine and dopamine are addictive; when we get in a "drug loop" in our brain, we can't think of anything but our next fix. Humans have a real problem with white powders that produce euphoria and craving—sugar and cocaine. We want more, more, more.

Whereas cocaine enhances good feelings, heroin and other narcotics, like Percocet and morphine, numb painful ones. We can think of an endorphin as internally produced morphine. A "runner's high" occurs when your body secretes endorphins in response to the "pain" of intense or long runs.

Certain foods, particularly those that have been altered genetically, contain exomorphins that act like pain relievers. One of the worst culprits is another deadly white powder—wheat flour. That's right; your hoagie roll has heroin-like properties. That's why many people reach for bread, pasta, and cookies as comfort foods. The exorphins those foods contain make the pain of the bad feelings go away—at least temporarily. Then withdrawal starts, and you start craving another "fix."

Although food is not actually a drug, once you ingest it, a huge array of chemicals is released in your brain. In fact, the simple act of thinking about food can cause massive amounts of "self-made" drugs to be released in your brain.

This process occurs in everybody—it's a part of the physiology that was essential to our survival as a species. For most of humankind's history, food wasn't necessarily very easy to acquire, and we needed the extra incentive provided by an internal chemical reward to pursue it. Humans are willing to work hard for things that may not be immediately available when we anticipate a reward at the end.

248

But in today's world, food is readily available; it requires so little work that we barely have to chew it! But our brains still compel us to seek reward, especially if we are stressed. So we engage in behaviors that stimulate production of those "self-made" drugs.

This is not the whole story, however. Our physiological well-being is geared towards trying to maintain equilibrium — homeostasis — and it is essential to our health and survival.

Our endogenous drugs are designed to help us maintain homeostasis. Exogenous drugs can easily upset this balance. Exogenous drugs stimulate your pleasure centers with unnatural intensity. Repeated exposures can lead to addiction; balance is lost and pleasure- or reward-seeking turns to pathological craving.

Modern-day food is highly stimulatory to our pleasure centers. One of the goals of the food industry is to chemically enhance foods so that they are more attractive to your pleasure centers, the same process used by the cigarette manufacturers to enhance the addictive properties of tobacco.

We are only beginning to understand that the food manufacturers are also employing this dangerous and destructive practice. When we eat a food that produces "self-made" drugs (all foods), and also contains "man-made drugs" (chemically altered food forgeries), that food emits a super-charged blast to the pleasure centers of our brain. These altered foods make us feel better, so we are much more likely to eat them again.

Real food is inherently rewarding, releasing endogenous neurochemicals, such as dopamine, endorphins, and serotonin (a "self-made" antidepressant and mood stabilizer). This is healthy and natural. It's the food forgeries that contain the "man-made" drugs that push us out of homeostasis, disrupt our natural pleasure centers, and make us become a slave to the crave.

One solution is to refer to the What skill, and to begin eating real food. Eating real food balances our hormones, sends the correct stimulation to our reward centers, and maintains our natural homeostatic rhythm. Another solution is to stop eating for stimulation, and begin eating for nourishment. That is our next *Evolutionary Eating* skill.

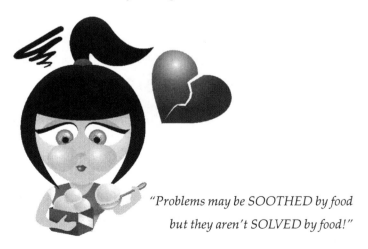

"Problems may be SOOTHED by food but they aren't SOLVED by food!"

The Solution

Learn the "WHY" Skill of Eating

Why do we eat? Why do we choose certain foods and avoid others? Why is it important to understand our eating behaviors, and our relationship with food? And why should we care? These are all important questions answered in the next *Evolutionary Eating* skill, called the "Why."

In the problem section, you learned that we are eating for stimulation instead of eating for nourishment. The reason Why we eat has changed.

This has had a dramatic effect on our health, happiness, and mental well-being—and particularly on our waistlines.

We've only begun this behavior of eating for stimulation quite recently, the primary reason being the highly stimulatory foodscape in which we currently live. The chemical-laden food forgeries give us a quick "high" that has hijacked our brains and our pleasure centers. We have become "junk-food junkies."

An important first step is to start eating real food — a skill outlined earlier in the book. You learned that our cells need nourishment and sustenance in the form of the building blocks and fuel we get from our digested food. Real food nourishes our cells, but human bodies also need to be nourished in other ways.

Traditionally and culturally, meals and food were the way we met our distinctly human spiritual, social, and celebratory needs. As our food culture has unraveled, it is not only the nutrients that have slipped through the cracks.

We are also suffering from a lack of that special form of nourishment that connects us as a group and grounds us as individuals. What we lack, we seek. We are hungry not just for the nourishment for our cells, but also for the nourishment of our souls.

Food should nourish us emotionally

Emotional eating is important because we are supposed to feel good when we eating. Skillful eaters are able to appreciate and savor what they are eating. They have positive emotions towards food.

Emotional overeaters are somewhat different. They eat for emotional reasons, but they often have negative emotions towards food. When they eat, they often feel guilty and ashamed. Many times, they eat not because they want the food, but because they want to mask an emotion. They eat for stimulation; they know that eating will give them that "quick-fix," just like a drug. So, one of the Why skills is to learn to enjoy our food instead of using it to avoid negative emotions.

Food is emotional, and it should nourish us emotionally. It should make us feel good, but it should not be used as a drug to temporarily avoid emotions that we need to deal with. Doing so is detrimental to our weight, health, and mental well-being.

Food should nourish us socially

Throughout human history, eating was the single most important activity for creating and developing social bonds.

Social nourishment is a vital component of our happiness and well-being. We are hardwired to want to be a part of a tribe because tribes had much better survival chances than single individuals.

The modern world has granted us more freedom and individual independence, but the need to be a part of a tribe is still there, etched into our genes.

In the past, food was always the primary activity for any group of people. From gathering and hunting, to preparing and cooking, and then finally eating, hours upon hours were spent devoted to the single activity of sharing food. We still have a craving for this social interaction, but we rarely get it today.

One of the ways our brains try to make up for this is by giving us cravings to eat. Eating has always been accompanied by people, and therefore our brains often make us want to eat when all we really need is social nourishment.

This is also why we watch so much TV. When we are socially malnourished, we try to find ways to compensate. TV provides us compensation because the primal parts of our brains do not recognize the difference between real people we interact with, and interactions that we watch on TV.

We can regain some of that social nourishment by referring to the When and Who skills. Eating meals with other people can be a tremendous opportunity to satisfy the normal human desire to connect with people.

Food should nourish us physically

We all know that we need food to survive. What many of us don't realize is that it is not enough to simply eat; we must eat the right type of foods that nourish and sustain our bodies.

Our body needs certain building blocks to function optimally. Past generations had a much easier time receiving the required building blocks because they ate food. This generation has had a much more difficult time because we are eating primarily food forgeries. When your body does not get what it needs, your brain will make you hungry. You can eat and eat and eat, but you will remain hungry.

Unfortunately, people who diet do not understand this fundamental principle at all. They think that they need to eat less, but all this does is provide their body with even fewer building blocks!!

If our food does not nourish us physically, then we nearly always overeat. That's just our brain's way of trying to get what it needs.

Food should nourish us intellectually

Food should not only nourish us emotionally, socially, and physically; it should also nourish us intellectually.

One way is learning about food. We are not born with knowledge about food; all we know is that we must eat. Learning about food preparation, cooking techniques, and new foods is extremely rewarding. There is great pleasure to be found in developing your taste buds, and enjoying new food experiences.

One of true joys of the table is the potential for meaningful conversation. Henry Wadsworth Longfellow summed it beautifully when he said, *"A single conversation across the table with a wise man is better than ten years' mere study of books."*

What can happen over the course of a meal is such a wonderful testament to our humanity. That's why we love the idea of feasts, and are so moved by movies like *My Dinner with Andre*, *Like Water for Chocolate*, and *Big Night*.

As with all necessary nourishment, when we don't get any intellectual stimulation, we look for it elsewhere. We become bored, agitated, and unhappy; in the end, we turn to the quick fix offered by the highly toxic, highly addictive non-food products that give us a drug-like fix. But it never lasts, and it's not long before we are back for more.

Eating for nourishment is a skill

When we eat for nourishment, we increase the pleasure that we receive from food, and thus we need to be stimulated less and less. This, of course, is a skill, and not something you can simply change overnight. You can't simply decide that you are no longer going to eat for stimulation. That's not how our habits and behaviors work.

Instead, what you need to do is to replace your eating for stimulation with a different activity. For example, if you always eat when you are bored, find an activity that gives you the same relief, but is a healthy behavior instead of a destructive one.

Getting support from skillful eaters may be among the best substitutions. Bonding over appreciating food, and appreciating being healthy is both beneficial and rewarding.

The "WHY" Skill of Eating

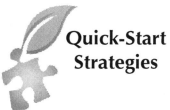 **Quick-Start Strategies**

It isn't particularly helpful to tell people to "reduce their stress." It's much more effective to have concrete strategies to avoid the overeating that often goes with stress, and to help you blunt the physiological effects of stress hormones on your health and wellness.

1) If you eat out of boredom, CUT IT OUT!

People who eat out of boredom are usually happy as long as what they eat fills up time, simply because they have nothing better to do.

The "cure" for eating out of boredom is planning. Find activities that occupy your mind, and do these instead of eating. It really is that simple, though yes, it does require planning. Be sure to have a list of at least three activities you can do instead of eating. The very act of being occupied is often enough for most people to eliminate this habit. By the way, this practice is much easier if you just enforce the "no-snacking" rule!

2) Stress will always be there—you can and should plan on it

In case you didn't know, increased levels of stress keep you stuck in fat-storage mode and the perpetual "gaining" cycle. Stress and stress hormones (which are what causes those "stress feelings") are a homeostatic response to perceived threat. Since your brain is blind, it doesn't know if the threat is real or imaginary, so it prepares you to deal with stress by dumping in hormones that will allow you to deal with danger in a physical way.

But in the modern world, most of our stress is mental and emotional. We never actually do anything, so we are stuck with the toxic leftovers of unused stress hormones that make us fat and hungry and, of course, "stressed out."

If you know that you have a stressful event in the future, write out exactly what you are going to eat. In fact, everybody should have a "stress plan," an eating plan that you always use under stressful situations.

3) Have an emergency meal—for emergencies!

Pack two "emergency meals." During stressful times, it is likely that you will not have time to prepare or buy healthy food, so you want to have two emergency meals available. These will replace the sugary snack that you would usually consume.

4) Avoid cues

Oscar Wilde said, *"The only way to get rid of temptation is to yield to it."* I recommend a different strategy: avoiding the stress of temptation whenever possible. To reduce impulsive indulgences, avoid walking past your local doughnut shop or the candy machine near your office.

We all have stress, and although it would be ideal to reduce your stress as much as possible, it is inevitable that such instances will occur. Plan for these occasions by using the strategies above or create some of your own.

5) Move more!

Bet you never thought I was going to mention exercise. Well, I'm a big fan of movement, as long as it's fun, invigorating, and not too stressful. I particularly like walking, vigorous play, and purposeful physical training. I like exercise that burns off stress hormones, not exercise that dumps in more (which is often what happens when people "go to the gym").

Most people use exercise as a substitute for movement, instead of a supplement. Human bodies need a lot of daily low-stress movement. I encourage you to first work on sitting less.

6) Nourish your body with REAL food

If your body is unwell because it is inflamed and toxic from too much rubbish, too much fuel, and not enough quality-building blocks, that is very stressful. Stress doesn't just come from the outside world. By definition, stress (or more accurately, "a stressor"), is anything that pushes you out of homeostasis. To decrease your stress, and enjoy the wonderful state of being what I call homeostatic hum, learn and practice the fundamental skills of eating.

7) Utilize non-food-related rewards

One of the major reasons that people overeat is simply because they use food as their primary reward. Instead, find alternative activities to reward yourself.

Some examples of simple rewards may be buying new clothes, getting a massage, playing with your dog, going to a movie, or whatever. It doesn't really matter as long as it is something that you enjoy.

8) Eliminate emotional overeating

Emotional overeating is usually about finding a way to instantly change the way you feel emotionally. That is why it almost always involves impulsive behaviors, like snacking, or bingeing on sweet, salty, and creamy foods.

If you can identify the pattern, you can change it. It usually includes a combination of the following factors: the same food, the same place, the same people, the same situations, the same time of day, the same quantities of food, the same mood, and the same reason.

Again, if you can establish under what situations emotional overeating occurs, you can develop strategies to either eliminate it, or to replace it with another behavior.

9) Understand your trigger behaviors, trigger times, and trigger situations

Triggers are environmental cues that create automatic and mindless eating. Once you understand your triggers, you can drastically reduce the amount of times you overeat.

Examples of trigger behaviors include nibbling, eating in front of the TV, consuming drinks and snacking in your car, and skipping meals and then overeating. Examples of trigger situations include overeating when you dine at restaurants, or always eating a certain type of food when it is available.

Examples of trigger times include any consistent times of day when you are susceptible to overeating. For most people, these times are in the late afternoon, in the evenings while waiting for dinner, or at the weekend when they are at home. It is vital that you identify these triggers. Doing so will allow you to eliminate some of your most detrimental eating habits.

10) Forget the last-meal syndrome

The last-meal syndrome is similar to the "my diet starts tomorrow" phenomena. This happens when you decide to binge so you can "eat it all" before you "start" your diet.

Stop fooling yourself! It will never be your last meal. If you have a piece of cake, then enjoy it. Don't eat the whole cake just because "this is the last time." (I really don't understand that cliché, "Having your cake and eating it too." Who would want to have cake that they couldn't eat?!)

11) Forget tomorrow

"My diet starts tomorrow"…"I'm beginning my new diet on Monday"…"My diet starts after I eat this"…Sound familiar?????

If you are reading this book, you are probably among the 99% of dieters who go on a diet, break their diet, and go on another diet, announcing, "My new diet starts tomorrow!" One of my favorite quotes is, *"The definition of insanity is trying the same thing over and over again, and expecting a different result."*

I really want you to stop this madness. Stop trying to fool yourself. There is no, "I'm starting my diet tomorrow." As soon as you say that, you have failed. The only diet is a *"diaeta"* —a way of life. So instead of starting your new diet tomorrow, start your new "way of life" RIGHT NOW. Remember, today is the first day of the rest of your life, not tomorrow. That is the only way you can change.

CHAPTER 8

"Are you ready to change for good?
If so, this book is the beginning
of your happily ever after."

The Problem

We Eat Like Babies,
So We Keep Growing (Wider)

The Solution

Grow Up

Now that you have ventured through the fundamental skills of eating, let's review where we started, and how far we have come.

When you picked up this book, you probably resembled a baby in many of your eating habits, but the wonderful thing about immaturity is that it's totally curable.

It's not too late to learn the fundamental skills of eating—it's never too late. Of course, this is a prime example of a problem that is simple, but not easy. Just because you understand the information doesn't mean you will apply it.

You can't learn a new skill, or especially a new habit, with a few repetitions — you must do it over and over again.

Recent bestsellers, like Malcolm Gladwell's, *Outliers*, and Geoff Colvin's, *Talent Is Overrated*, point out how important it is to repeat new behaviors over and over again, with deliberate attention. That is the only way to extinguish the old habit and replace it with a new-and-improved version.

Adults can learn the skills of eating in a much shorter time than children by practicing with awareness and intention. But children don't need to unlearn old habits, so these new behaviors will not happen automatically.

Though I wish it were otherwise, they also won't happen even if you have a great Aha! moment while reading this book. It's simply not the way our brain works. It seems like our brain should care about what we think, but it really doesn't. Our brain only cares about what we do, and what we must do is change.

This book is about changing for good. It really is your chance to a happily ever after. Maybe that sounds good to you, or maybe it sounds good, but not just yet.

A lot of people want to do things in the future, when they have some time. I want to remind you that you've already got all the time there is. There isn't any more. You have the same amount as everyone else — 24 hours a day. How you choose to use it is your decision. It is not the time, but what you do with it, that counts.

Often, people think they fail at something because they don't have the time or money. But I don't believe that's true. It's amazing what people can do with no time or money when they feel supported.

That's why I wrote this book.

I want you to be successful.
Make sure you have enough support.
You are not alone.

Reach for a hand, and reach out a hand—that's what makes it all worthwhile. I feel confident that because you are a human, and therefore capable of extraordinary feats of learning and skill development, you will begin to make the kind of changes in your behavior that signal the end of booty camp, and the start of your happily ever after.

The Quick, Quick, Quick Strategies!

I put the high-payoff quick strategies here. Once you have read the book, you will understand why these are so helpful. But some people (like me, for example) always peek at the end first. So here they are, broken down by skill.

WHEN to eat

⬛ Eat regular meals.

⬛ Eat no more than three meals a day.

⬛ Try to eat on schedule; it will optimize hunger hormones faster.

⬛ Don't eat for at least two to three hours before bedtime.

⬛ Don't snack.

⬛ DON'T SNACK.

WHAT to eat

Learn the difference between real food and food forgeries.

Shop on the perimeter of the grocery store; that's where the real food usually is.

Avoid sweets, except for planned-in-advance special occasions.

Limit your carbohydrates to decrease insulin resistance; that means avoid starches, like bread, pasta, or cereal.

Keep cutting back on processed food.

Avoid industrially produced oils and products that use them, such as salad dressings and processed food.

Replace "vegetable oils" with healthy oils and fats, like olive oil, butter, and coconut oil.

Eat colorful, fresh vegetables, preferably organic.

Eat meat products from animals raised in a humane and healthy way; remember you are eating "what they ate."

WHERE to eat

Eat at a designated place at home, preferably a table.

When you eat outside the home, also choose a designated spot.

Make, and enforce, Food-Free ZONES, like the car, and the bedroom.

If you eat in front of the TV, treat it like a meal, not a munch out.

Plan and prepare your food—restaurants are tricky unless you are a skillful eater!

Have two emergency meals on hand—for emergencies!

DON'T DRINK YOUR FUEL! There are no caloric beverages in nature.

WHO to eat with

Identify and avoid saboteurs, especially at mealtimes!

Pretend you are eating with a virtual companion who has excellent food skills.

⟋ Understand that all humans are susceptible to media images that deal with people and eating behavior.

⟋ Prepare a list of canned excuses, like "I have a food allergy."

⟋ Even better, practice saying aloud, "No, thank you. I don't like to eat when I'm not hungry."

HOW to eat

⟋ Eat your food from a 9-inch plate that has a border. (Un-supersize your cutlery, bowls, etc., at the same time.)

⟋ Serve up your plate in the kitchen, so you really have to consider whether you want to have seconds.

⟋ Make a mental speed bump halfway through your meal, "Do I want to eat more?"

⟋ Chew your food, and choose food that requires chewing!

⟋ Use utensils and (audible gasp) "table manners."

⟋ Use tall, thin glasses.

WHY to eat

🌿 Recognize when a binge is building; distract yourself.

🌿 Learn a new skill that you can practice when you are bored and hungry.

🌿 Avoid mindless eating—keep food out of sight.

🌿 Habitats make habits. If it's in the house, you'll eat it... get tempting food out of the house.

🌿 Don't beat yourself up for backsliding. This is a program for life. Life is full of stumbles. Life goes on.

*You and I, dear reader,
started with a once upon a time
of the modern world.*

*We end with a happily ever after:
your happily ever after.*

*Thank you for your attention.
Theresa*

36305225R00156

Made in the USA
San Bernardino, CA
19 July 2016